Success Stories and Results

'Michelle's advice, guidance and meal plan have helped me lose an amazing amount of weight, without feeling hungry and with significant benefits to my health and well-being. I love her recipes, which I make for my whole family (including three ravenous sons), who don't even realise I'm on a diet'   *Elizabeth*, barrister

'Michelle didn't put me on a diet, she taught me the value of healthy eating through The Food Effect approach and principles. Food and cooking have been transformed from being a burden to being fun, colourful, exciting and delicious. It is not an exaggeration to say that Michelle has literally changed my life – and the inside of my fridge and larder'   *Stacey*, retail consultant

'Michelle is such a great coach. Everyone should have a Michelle in their life'   *Liz*, charity director

'I went to see Michelle primarily because I needed help controlling some long-standing stomach issues. Michelle suggested The Food Effect diet plan, which was easy to follow and allowed me to eat much more than I was eating before, but this time to eat the correct foods. Within a week my stomach symptoms were under control and I was losing weight, too. In four months I lost 8kg, and the best part is that I no longer take any medication for my stomach. Michelle – I was sceptical at first about eating more and losing weight, but guess what? You were right. Thank you for turning my life around'   *Esther*, psychologist and teacher

'Through living and eating The Food Effect way, Michelle shows that food can be healthy and enjoyable at the same time. The meals and recipes are outstanding, colourful and delicious, and about as far from dullness and deprivation as I could imagine'
     Gemma, accountant

'Having adopted vegetarianism at seven years old, I was never really overweight even though I didn't eat particularly healthily. That all changed when I got married at twenty-four. The weight slowly crept on as I gave in to all sorts of bad cravings – copious amounts of refined carbs in many forms, unhealthy processed 'vegetarian' products, and many sugary treats were the order of the day, quite literally. At the time of going to see Michelle, I weighed in at 93kg and needed to lose about 23kg of that (to get to my optimal weight of 70kg). I did a lot of research and came across Dr Michelle Braude and The Food Effect through acquaintances who couldn't recommend her more highly. With her combined medical knowledge and expertise in nutrition, I felt so at ease with the meal plan and lifestyle she prescribed for me. I loved that I was able to share my blood results with Michelle (charted all the way through my weight-loss journey), and I have my blood pressure taken at every follow-up. Today, three years later, I weigh 68kg thanks to The Food Effect way of living. I have kept a consistent weight to what I got to with Michelle (with a slight fluctuation of up to 2kg maximum) and have never been happier. What Michelle does is lifesaving stuff. I cannot thank her enough'   *David*, IT consultant

'Michelle was outstanding in educating me and helping me see that I didn't have to refrain from eating everything I loved to achieve a healthy, slimmer me. I have lost 10kg and kept it off, and I am still having my beloved fried egg sandwich on a Friday morning, which The Food Effect diet allows. I feel better than I have in many years'

Trevor, banker and senior relationship manager

'I went to see Michelle precisely because she is medically qualified – I truly believe that someone who influences my diet needs to have a holistic approach, and only someone medically as well as nutritionally qualified has the ability to do that. I'm a challenging case because I'm vegetarian and have lots of food fads, which means I have a pretty restricted diet. Nevertheless,

Michelle was able to design a diet for me that I've been able to follow and stick to, since seeing her originally now several years ago. The Food Effect really is a way of life. I went to see her weighing 95kg, and several months later I was down to 83kg and have kept the weight off. I could still do with shedding quite a few kilograms more, and thanks to Michelle I know exactly how to do that. It's just a question of how disciplined I am in following The Food Effect plan, which really is so simple and manageable. I have no excuse'

Mark, communications company owner

'The Food Effect diet has transformed my life. I love my eating plan and look forward to my meals and snacks. I am never hungry and am still losing weight. Thanks Michelle'

Judy, personal assistant

'Thank you to Michelle at The Food Effect for such inspirational, healthy and delicious recipes and meal ideas for the busy professional. For me, as a busy doctor who never stops, they make eating well extremely possible' *Daniel*, anaesthetist

THE
FOOD
EFFECT
DIET

DR MICHELLE BRAUDE

piatkus

PIATKUS

First published in Great Britain in 2017 by Piatkus

1 3 5 7 9 10 8 6 4 2

A CIP catalogue record for this book
is available from the British Library.

ISBN 978-0-349-41582-6

Typeset in Sabon by M Rules
Printed and bound in Great Britain by
Clays Ltd, St Ives plc

Papers used by Piatkus are from well-managed forests
and other responsible sources.

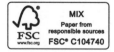

Piatkus
An imprint of
Little, Brown Book Group
Carmelite House
50 Victoria Embankment
London EC4Y 0DZ

An Hachette UK Company
www.hachette.co.uk

www.improvementzone.co.uk

Dedicated to my husband Jeff —
the love of my life and wind beneath my wings

ABOUT THE AUTHOR

A qualified medical doctor and nutritionist who founded The Food Effect, www.thefoodeffect.co.uk, Dr Michelle Braude runs an innovative nutrition consultancy practice based in north London, as well as a popular online blog in which she shares and explains the health benefits of her favourite recipes.

Born in sunny South Africa and raised in London, Michelle is at the forefront of the future of healthcare. She combines her background in medicine, expertise in the science of nutrition, and passion for cooking and good food, to offer a comprehensive and practical service that is unique.

Michelle qualified as a medical doctor (MBBS) from the prestigious University College London (UCL). During her medical studies, she completed a Bachelor of Science (BSc) degree in nutrition at King's College London, as well as carrying out an elective period in gastroenterology at the Whittington Hospital, London. This provided further opportunity for her to increase her knowledge and gain practical experience in the wide range of clinical conditions covered by this area of medicine.

Not long after graduating, Michelle's passion for nutrition prompted her to set up her own practice, The Food Effect, in 2012. With mounting clinical evidence of the effect of nutrition on health and well-being, Michelle realised she could use her combined knowledge in the fields of medicine and nutrition to help patients with medical conditions, such as high blood pressure, high cholesterol and diabetes, to improve their health through their diets. As her unique approach developed, she also began specialising in improving the diets and optimising the overall health and well-being of people who did not have a medical condition but needed to lose weight. Within a year, the project had become a hugely successful nutrition practice and online business. Needless to say, the next logical step was to share her secrets in a book.

Since officially founding The Food Effect, Michelle's reputation and practice have grown rapidly. Her unique expertise in the field of nutrition, teamed with her growing public and online profiles, have resulted in Michelle being a sought-after expert. She is regularly featured as an independent expert in the *Daily Mail*, the *Telegraph, Hello!, Women's Health*, the *Mirror, Marie Claire*, and *LOOK* magazine. She is also a regular writer for the hugely successful international luxury web magazine *Chic Overdose*, popular models' website *Modellist-ID* and medical experts' website *Good Zing*, and Byrdie Beauty UK.

CONTENTS

The Food Effect diet – eat more, weigh less, look better and feel better

Ditch the fad diets, juice cleanses, 'detoxes' and all the other crazes out there. That's the message of The Food Effect approach to nutrition – which, based on real science, separates the facts from the fads.

Most people who lose weight through dieting do *not* keep the weight off in the long term. This is certainly something I have seen with countless desperate clients who were in this position until they adopted The Food Effect approach and have since never looked back – or put the weight back on.

People try the latest fad diet or follow advice to cut out certain food groups, stick to it for a few weeks or months, and drop some pounds, but sooner or later they 'come off' the diet and return to their old eating habits. They regain the weight – and possibly increase it – and when the next 'miracle' diet comes along, they start the whole disheartening process again. Most diets fail because they are overly restrictive and mind-numbingly lacking in variety. This makes it impossible to stick to these diets in the long term.

At the other end of the spectrum is the 'clean-eating' brigade, whose beautiful recipe books are filled with pictures of avocado toast liberally drizzled with olive oil, and smoothie bowls with rainbow-striped toppings or a smiley face of chia seeds, but whose advice is often not based on any scientific knowledge or facts. Most worryingly, while such meals and snacks might be delicious, they can in fact rack up a huge amount of calories. If people follow such diets in the naïve assumption that everything 'healthy' equates with 'not fattening' (without the need to spend all day in the gym), this will in fact lead to an excess calorie intake and weight gain. Porridge topped with coconut oil, chopped nuts, cacao nibs, chia seeds, almond butter and agave syrup may well be delicious, but eating it regularly is likely to sabotage any weight-loss efforts and may well lead to weight gain in the long term.

Bearing this in mind, The Food Effect philosophy grew from my desire to teach people how to eat normally and healthily in a way that can continue for the rest of their lives. It is based on the belief that healthy eating is an essential, pleasurable, colourful and vibrant way of life – and one that can be achieved by everyone, if they are shown how.

In the course of building up a successful practice, and treating hundreds of happy clients, I developed the Food Effect diet and lifestyle plan to show you how you can eat more, weigh less and both look and feel better – without compromising your lifestyle.

The Food Effect Diet presents a simple, delicious and satisfying way of eating that sheds weight, boosts energy, lowers cholesterol and blood pressure, and gives you glowing skin, increased brain power and optimal health and vitality. It teaches the simple secrets of long-term practical success for weight loss, but it does not require you to cut out any foods groups or do any specific exercise. Instead, you'll be encouraged to eat carbs at every meal, have a late-night treat and avoid the faddish route of cutting out wheat, gluten, dairy, carbs or fats. What's more, you'll be allowed to dine out and enjoy coffee, alcohol and chocolate from day one – without it compromising your weight-loss goals.

The Food Effect diet encompasses:

- Two simple stages (the Food Effect attack phase and Food Effect lifestyle phase) that are incredibly easy to stick to.
- A wide array of food choices, including surprising sources of 'good for you' carbs.
- Menu options for breakfast, lunch, dinner and snacks based on a variety of taste preferences, lifestyles and nutritional needs.
- Sixty-five delicious and easy recipes, plus a complete set of simple meal ideas for those who don't like to cook, or don't have time to do so.
- Practical, comprehensive food tables, featuring every food group (from proteins, carbs, fruit and vegetables, to beverages, condiments and alcohol), in clear, practical 'eat this', 'be careful' and 'stay away' categories.
- Dietary recommendations – designed with a calorie cap (so there's no calorie counting involved) to ensure you achieve your weight-loss goals.
- Plenty of variety to keep things interesting.
- Up-to-the minute tips and advice, including supplement advice and recommendations (this is much more straightforward than you think).
- Advice on overcoming potential obstacles and common challenges, including tips on managing cravings and overeating.

These days, we seem to be gluttons for fad diets, but while they may appear to be a 'quick-fix solution' and lead to weight loss in the short term, over time they slow down your metabolism, are unsustainable and simply cause you to pile the pounds back on straight after you come off them.

The Food Effect approach, in contrast, is based on scientific understanding of anatomy and physiology, and doesn't change with the tides of fad dieting, juice cleanses, soup diets or detoxes.

In this book, I share the simple strategies that I have used to help hundreds of clients shed weight and – more importantly – keep it off, while at the same time improving their health, energy and vitality.

So what sets my plan apart from the current swathe of trendy fad diets? There two major differences:

1. It is nutritionally sound.
2. It has earned the approval of medical experts and dieters alike.

Simple and effective without being overly complicated, The Food Effect diet delivers a painless and proven way to achieve your weight-loss goals and get you on the road to optimal health. It's all about eating more of the right things. That means packing in as much good, wholesome nutrition as possible via delicious healthy meals and snacks so that there's no room for the bad stuff.

What's more, by eating delicious, wholesome, tasty foods (not dry tuna and lettuce leaves) you won't find it difficult to stick to, either, and you certainly won't be expected to go hungry. It's all about making simple changes that don't feel like a sacrifice – for example, swapping crisps for salted popcorn, or switching from unhealthy processed puddings and biscuits to far healthier dark chocolate or guilt-free Greek yoghurt with fruit for dessert. That way you won't ever feel as though you're missing out.

The Food Effect diet – what makes it unique?

The Food Effect approach is a revolutionary concept in weight loss, weight management and healthy living. As a self-confessed 'foodie' – as well as a medical doctor with a degree in nutrition – I'm confident in the unique strengths of The Food Effect system, which are based on the combination of the three key areas of science, choice and taste.

Science: medical and scientific knowledge All the advice in this book is based on a thorough understanding of nutritional science and constant engagement with the latest developments in the world of nutrition. It is combined with a comprehensive understanding of health and medical conditions, which I gained through my studies and strive to maintain, ensuring that all advice for weight loss addresses nutritional needs in the most holistic and optimal way.

Choice: tailored solutions I strive to fully appreciate and encompass different lifestyles and eating preferences so that the advice in this book is workable and can be tailored by you to suit your individual needs. In addition to being nutritionally comprehensive, The Food Effect advice is simple, practical and realistic, ensuring the optimum chance of success.

Taste: culinary passion and expertise I'm passionate about food and cooking, and fully appreciate that you want to enjoy your food, so I channel this understanding into all my advice to ensure that the meal plans I provide are both varied and tasty. In addition, I have included useful shopping guides, delicious recipes, and healthy cooking and dining-out advice. Together, these resources will help you every step along the way as you discover that a healthy weight-loss diet can be both enjoyable and effective.

The combination of science, choice and great tastes makes this a comprehensive approach to weight loss and greater well-being. You will become more knowledgeable about healthy eating in a way that helps you lead a happier, healthier life – all while looking and feeling great. Best of all, you will achieve all of this while still enjoying your food and losing weight. It's a distinctive approach that has shown phenomenal results over the past few years with my growing client base, who have all embraced The Food Effect way of eating and living – and never looked back.

The Food Effect diet is not low carb; nor is it low fat. It teaches you to rely on the *right* carbs and the *right* fats, combined with the best proteins, while avoiding the wrong things – and shows you how to live very happily without them. As a result, you get healthy and lose weight – around 6–12lb in the first four weeks alone (during The Food Effect attack phase), and thereafter 1–2lb a week (following The Food Effect lifestyle) until you reach your goal weight. (The exact amount you lose will depend on how much weight you have to lose – the more excess weight you're carrying, the more you can expect to lose.) Better yet, your new way of eating and The Food Effect lifestyle will ensure that the weight stays off – so that you get slim and *stay* slim.

You'll do this by eating normal-sized helpings of chicken, turkey, fish, dairy foods, nuts and eggs, combined with ample good carbohydrates and fats. You'll have plenty of fruit and vegetables, with no nonsense telling you that you should cut out fruit because it has too much sugar in it, or that you need to go dairy- and gluten-free. You will need to cut out red meat (lamb, beef, pork) initially, but you'll be allowed coffee, dairy foods, carbs, chocolate and alcohol from day one. The science behind all this will be explained.

You'll eat three balanced meals a day, as well as two healthy and enjoyable snacks. Everything in the plan is designed so that you won't go hungry. Nothing undermines a weight-loss programme more than the distressing sensation of feeling unsatisfied and hungry – which inevitably ends in bingeing or the need to 'break' the diet. On The Food Effect plan you will have a snack mid-afternoon, whether you feel hungry or not. You'll also have a treat every night at whatever time you wish, be it after dinner or at midnight.

If you're the kind of person who 'lives for' bread, pasta and carbs, you won't have to give them up; and if you're the type that can't get through the day without a sugary chocolate bar, sweets or crisps, this plan is going to painlessly help you ditch those urges and cravings for good. It might be challenging for the first day or two, but by cleverly including the *right* carbohydrates, perfectly designed meals and snacks, and an evening treat, you won't have such a hard time fighting your urges. Within a few days, your cravings will disappear. I can say this with confidence because I've seen it with so many overweight people, unhealthy eaters and sugar- or junk-food addicts who have succeeded on The Food Effect programme. There's also a whole chapter of tips and tricks for helping you to manage cravings and avoid overeating. The Food Effect diet may be new 'on the shelves', but it has existed for several years – long enough to have helped hundreds of my clients lose weight with ease, and keep it off.

Many diets, nutrition plans, cleanses and 'detoxes' will enable you to lose weight, but leave you with dull, lifeless skin, lacking in energy, and often feeling hungry, tired, dizzy and even faint. Not only are such diets inadvisable from a health perspective, but they are unsustainable. In contrast, The Food Effect lifestyle plan recognises that weight loss is just one benefit of healthy eating. When properly planned to include all the key nutrients, what we eat has a dramatic impact on how we look, feel and function. A diet should aspire to achieve all of that – weight loss should not come at the expense of overall health and optimal physical functioning.

When it comes to sustainability, the benefit of The Food Effect lifestyle is that it is self-reinforcing. The more we eat in a wholesome way, the better we look and feel, and the more we *want* to eat in a wholesome way. Our bodies adapt to an optimum weight, our biological systems improve and we find ourselves full of the energy that lies dormant inside every one of us. You will quite literally feel The Food Effect. A diet like this then ceases to be a diet, and instead becomes a fully fledged way of life.

Developing a healthy-eating lifestyle

The three elements involved in developing a healthy-eating life-style are simplicity, pleasure and sustainability.

Simplicity

Achieving proper nutrition can be confusing for two reasons. The myriad of fad diets, unproven practices and conflicting nutritional information that we are presented with daily in books and magazines, online and on TV can cloud our ability to properly understand what is (and is not) good for us. Even some healthy diets are overly complicated due to the inclusion of obscure and overpriced products that are entirely unnecessary for a healthy, balanced diet.

With a thorough understanding of both the human body and the science of nutrition, it is possible to create a diet that is nutritionally complete in accordance with proven science, as well as being simple. I know this is the case, because that is pre-cisely what I have created with The Food Effect diet. Simplicity means that the diet is not complicated or expensive, but rather made up of ingredients available in every local supermarket at reasonable prices. Simplicity also means that putting the diet into practice is not time-consuming – there is no reason why 'no time' or 'too busy' should ever be an excuse for unhealthy eating.

Healthy eating should be easily achievable for everyone – from busy parents at home to high-flying, frequently flying corporate executives; for those looking to simply lose weight and feel better, to those with chronic medical conditions who want to improve their symptoms and overall health. The Food Effect programme makes all this possible irrespective of your circumstances.

Pleasure

Food is unavoidably a central part of our daily lives. A diet should not be something we 'go on' and 'go off', but rather a way of life. In keeping with this, our food should be delicious and leave us feeling satisfied – not hungry and deprived. The focus of a diet should not only be on what to *exclude*, but more importantly on what to *include*. The elimination of entire food groups, calorie counting and complicated instructions result in eating becoming a chore rather than a pleasure. This inevitably ends with you asking when you can come off the diet and eat all the things you miss again.

Through sensible changes, The Food Effect diet will show you that eating in a healthy, wholesome way is tremendously pleasurable. You will enjoy the textures and tastes found in abundance across *all* the food groups. You will find yourself enjoying eating and feeling full, and your body will respond in kind – absorbing plenty of nutrients from a variety of sources and becoming slim. To achieve all of this is something that appears unachievable in the standard Western diet, yet in reality it's so simple.

Sustainability

It is self-evident that if a diet is going to work and result in a change in our habits, it has to be sustainable, otherwise any benefits achieved will soon be lost. Incorporating all the elements described above – creating a properly designed nutrition plan that keeps things simple and pleasurable – makes lifelong change achievable for everyone.

Once you learn to eat this way, you won't want to go back – it's a change for life.

CHAPTER 1

My Story

From neurosurgeon to nutritionist – and my message to you

OK, so I was never a neurosurgeon, but for many years that was much closer to the path I was on than the one I am on now. An ambitious academic child who always wanted to be 'a TV presenter or surgeon' (as expressed in my primary school, thereby gaining many adult laughs), I did in fact pursue my dream of becoming a qualified medical doctor at the prestigious University College London (UCL), much to my dad's delight.

Yet I've also always loved all things health, food and nutrition; I find the science behind it fascinating and am forever challenged and intrigued by what drives us to make certain food choices. Born in sunny South Africa, where healthy eating and good food are a way of life, I've also always had a passion for cooking. My mum is one of the best cooks I know, and I've grown up watching her create the most delicious meals (and enjoying eating them, too). I grew up eating healthy, wholesome, nutritious food without being deprived of anything or given the message that certain foods should be restricted. Meals were packed with protein, whole-grain carbohydrates, healthy fats (avocados are a staple in South Africa), fruit and vegetables. I loved salads and everything healthy, but there was always chocolate in the cupboard and my mum baked cakes and biscuits regularly.

I was allowed to feel comfortable around food, knowing that if I wanted to eat a piece of cake as a treat, that was OK and I wouldn't wake up fat. At the same time, however, I was 'shown' in an indirect way that healthy food was 'nicer' and so much better for me than unhealthy food and, in fact, I enjoyed it more. I loved feeling full, satisfied and energised due to eating hearty, wholesome meals. The chocolate often remained untouched in the cupboard because I didn't feel that I 'needed' it. That's what happens when healthy eating becomes a way of life rather than something restrictive that is associated with dullness and deprivation, which ultimately leads to cravings and binges (more on that in Chapter 7).

Thankfully, the balance I was taught from an early age carried me through my teenage years and young adult life – when I finally decided to hang up the white coat and to start my work as a nutritionist at The Food Effect, my own innovative nutrition consultancy practice and, later, popular online blog (at www.thefoodeffect.co.uk). I continue to share my ideas with my clients and followers today, and teach people – through the understanding that healthy eating is actually so much simpler than we're led to believe – how to eat better. I'm so grateful to be able to combine my passion for healthy eating with my knowledge of nutrition and love of interesting new recipes, in order to create wonderfully delicious (yet simple) meals. This has been a key element in creating The Food Effect diet. It really is a way of life, and one that I'm excited to be sharing with you.

How The Food Effect came to be

Despite realising early on that medicine may not be quite the right path for me, I plodded along, spending days (and nights) in hospitals, ditching sleep in favour of revising for endless exams.

During this time, however, I also completed a degree in nutrition at King's College London, which only deepened the chasm between what I was doing and what I felt I should be doing.

More and more over the course of my last few years as a burnt-out medical student, I realised that I didn't want to spend the rest of my career working as a hospital doctor, but that I still wanted to use the knowledge I had gained from studying medicine and continue to work in a medically related field, perhaps combining this with my passion for nutrition and the BSc I had gained in it.

Doctors should prescribe nuts, olive oil and vegetables

I finally had a 'light-bulb moment' during a GP placement in my final year of medicine.

That moment came at a point when I had already begun to get extremely frustrated at seeing heart attack patients who had just had bypass surgery being served fried fish and chips in their hospital beds. I also saw hugely overweight men coming to see their GP, having been newly diagnosed with high blood pressure or high cholesterol (or both), and simply being handed an ongoing prescription for drugs such as statins, without *any* lifestyle or dietary advice, or even being told to lose weight. I was shocked and appalled.

It angered and frustrated me how little emphasis was put on diet in everyday medical settings. Thankfully, our society is now becoming aware of the importance of healthy eating, and the fact that doctors often fail to 'prescribe' it is something that's now drawing headline news. A large number of people are overweight, depressed, diabetic and have a high risk of heart disease because many doctors are inept at providing effective dietary information to their patients. Experts at a 2016 international health conference at the Royal Society of Medicine in London highlighted that the lack of nutritional education available to medical staff amounted to clinical negligence.

Fortunately, I realised this myself back in 2011, and it gave me the impetus I needed to review my career and follow my passion. At the time I was doing my student placement at a GP practice and was assessing a fifteen-year-old girl who came in with weakness, exhaustion and shortness of breath. Nothing the doctor had suggested on previous visits had helped her or provided any avenues to explore, and her exhaustion was getting worse and worse. I was given ten minutes alone with the girl to take a brief medical history. I asked her about her menstrual periods, whether she had ever had her iron levels checked and what her current diet was like. In short, this young girl had lost her parents at an early age, lived with her elderly grandmother, who she took care of, and there was no one doing any cooking or food shopping for her. She told me about her very heavy periods and described her daily diet, which consisted of nothing more than white bread or toast, plain white pasta and bags of crisps in between. When I asked her if she ate any fruit or vegetables, or fish, meat, dairy foods or any other forms of protein at all, she told me 'never', the reason being that they were more expensive than her current staples. Even more shocking was the fact that she didn't see anything wrong with this, or realise the importance of those essential basic food groups – not to mention the admission that no doctor had ever asked her about her diet on previous visits. After discussing her diet and nutrition in more detail, it was clear to me that the solution lay in improving it. This episode finally gave me the conviction I needed; expert nutritional advice from a doctor would not just be helpful but *essential* in future healthcare. Moreover, I knew I had to build on this idea.

This episode pushed me to take a year out from hospital medicine soon after graduating, and do something about my passion for nutrition. Thus The Food Effect nutrition practice was born. In short, my 'crazy' idea, which I planned to do for only a year, went on to become a hugely busy and successful nutrition practice and online blog, all of which I run myself, with my dad – who was initially concerned about my switch from 'surgeon' to nutritionist – now being my guiding rock and greatest supporter.

Starting out

Of course, I never dreamt that my 'little business' for my year out of clinical practice could become a long-term career. Starting my own business, however, was no easy feat. I had to learn everything from scratch. I'd spent all my years since school either as a medical student or in an NHS hospital – I had absolutely no idea about anything commercial or business related, so I simply gave it a go and learnt along the way.

While I'll never go back to clinical medicine, I'm grateful that I get to see plenty of interesting cases – often clients come to me who have co-existent conditions and are on a range of medications, so my medical knowledge is put to use on a daily basis and was certainly paramount in developing The Food Effect diet.

All my clients – from day one – have been my motivation, and ultimately what led me to write this book. I feel incredibly satisfied when clients report that The Food Effect way of eating has changed their lives on so many levels – improved health, energy, better relationships, looking and feeling better, and loving life more. I am blessed to have the opportunity to help so many people in a field that is so undervalued in our society and healthcare system.

What I've learnt and what I'd like to pass on to you

The attributes I developed in becoming a doctor have no doubt helped tremendously in my career as a nutritionist. They include empathy for others, being used to hard work and long hours, and appreciating the importance of patient confidentiality. In addition, everything I learnt in my years studying has given me an in-depth knowledge and appreciation for every aspect of the human body, which is hugely beneficial to my career in an area where very few (if any) nutritionists are qualified doctors.

Despite my convictions, I had a hard time for a few months when making the switch. Worrying about what others thought of my decision, feeling I had let my parents down and having to explain to everyone I saw or spoke to that I was not carrying on with medicine was definitely the most challenging aspect of my career transition.

However, every cloud has a silver lining, as they say. In my case, the struggle to change career has given me the great advantage of knowing how to motivate people who may otherwise lack the support and encouragement that is required in the journey towards healthy eating and optimal living. The bottom line is: never let the naysayers get in your way – no matter what anyone thinks or however much people try to put you off. If I had done so, I'd probably still be stuck in a job that wasn't making me feel good about myself because it simply wasn't the right fit for me. Instead – since leaving medicine – my confidence has soared and I feel happier and more fulfilled, as you will, too, once you've adopted the lifestyle changes I suggest and start to achieve your health and weight-loss goals. After all, no one should be stuck in a body that doesn't make them feel good – no matter what anyone says.

Work hard and give everything you do 100 per cent effort because you only get out what you put in. My message to you is that you should 'go for it' and work hard. If you never try, you'll never know. This applies to everything, from work and business to healthy eating and living.

Confidence also plays a huge role in success in any pursuit – you don't need to be perfect, but if you believe you can do something, you will succeed. So start this book with a positive outlook and throw any negative thoughts out the window now.

There's no place for 'I can't do this', or 'it won't work for me because of xyz ...' If you make excuses, there'll always be a reason why now is not the right time. That's a key message of The Food Effect diet – don't settle for an unhappy, mediocre version of yourself when you can look and feel the best you can be.

If you face mental or emotional obstacles when embarking on this new way of life, hopefully the words of the famous quote from Marianne Williamson's book *A Return to Love*, will inspire you:

> Our deepest fear is not that we are inadequate. Our deepest fear is that we are powerful beyond measure. It is our light, not our darkness that most frightens us. We ask ourselves, 'Who am I to be brilliant, gorgeous, talented and fabulous?' Actually, who are you not to be?

Who are you not to be brilliant, gorgeous, talented and fabulous – in a body that you feel amazing in? Yes, there are those who may try to put you off, but remember that their attitude may be born out of a fear of their own inability to change and uncertainty as to the potential that lies within you. However, just imagine the positive knock-on effects of embarking on such life-enhancing changes, for those around you, as well as yourself. The possibilities really are endless.

*

Thus, with some little personal anecdotes from me, a whole host of reasons for joining the journey that you simply cannot refute, and a tiny taster of what this exciting new lifestyle has in store for you, you're ready to move on to Chapter 2, which is all about getting started and understanding The Food Effect diet.

CHAPTER 2

Getting Started

Understanding The Food Effect diet

With so much to gain, it's understandable that by now you're probably eager to begin The Food Effect diet, in order to experience 'The Food Effect' for yourself. By doing so, you will begin a journey that will not only help you lose weight, but will also enhance your overall health, vitality and longevity.

The first step is to follow phase one, The Food Effect 28-day attack phase, before moving on to phase two, The Food Effect lifestyle. These are discussed further in this chapter, and in a lot more detail with the meal options and plans laid out in full in Chapters 11 and 12.

Before you start the programme, you need some basic information on what to eat – and what to avoid. This is provided in the tables on the effects of food on health and weight that follow in this chapter, as well as the key guidelines laid out in the rules and tips for healthy eating and weight loss (see pages 28 and 30).

Chapters 3 to 10 provide you with essential knowledge you need to understand the rationale behind The Food Effect approach; as the saying goes, 'knowledge is power', so don't skip these. They also provide a wealth of tips and tricks on everything from dining out healthily and drinking alcohol, to snacking smartly and banishing cravings.

Once you begin this programme, you will never look at food and eating in the same way again. You will still enjoy food and love to eat, but you will do so with an appreciation and understanding that you probably didn't have before. There will be no more hunger or deprivation, and no more fad diets. The Food Effect is about finally learning how to lose weight while eating a well-balanced diet for the rest of your life.

Chapters 3, 4, 5 and 6 provide valuable information about carbohydrates, protein and fats: which ones you're going to be eating, and what you'll be avoiding and why. But first, this chapter outlines the foods you can and can't eat. It couldn't be easier.

The eat-this, be-careful and stay-away tables

In this section you will find all the food groups (fruit, vegetables, legumes, fats and oils, nuts and seeds, grains and carbohydrates, proteins, dairy foods and alternatives, beverages and condiments) laid out in tables, divided into 'eat this', 'be careful' and 'stay away' columns to make knowing what to eat and what to avoid simple and effortless. Once you've looked at the tables a few times, you probably won't need to look back at them often. As I've stressed, The Food Effect way of eating becomes a lifestyle rather than a diet.

The titles at the tops of the columns are pretty self-explanatory, and while I wouldn't advocate that you never have a piece of cake again (after all, what's a birthday without some cake?), as a general rule 'stay away' means exactly that, as all the foods listed under this column do absolutely nothing to benefit your health or weight, and will just prevent you achieving your weight-loss goals. 'Be careful' might mean 'consume in moderation', as in the case of low-fat mayonnaise or Manuka honey, or alternatively that a food is not the best option but is not 'terrible', so you can have it occasionally (such foods include white rice, white potatoes and white pasta), if that's all that's available, for example when dining out.

By eating The Food Effect way, made easy with these tables, you'll get healthy and lose weight – around 6–12lb in the first four weeks alone (during the attack phase), and thereafter 1–2lb a week (following the lifestyle phase), until you reach your goal weight. (As mentioned earlier, the exact amount of weight you lose will vary according to how much you need to lose – the more excess weight you're carrying, the more you can expect to lose.) Better yet, your new way of eating and The Food Effect lifestyle will ensure that the weight stays off – so as well as getting slim you'll stay slim.

When cooking at home, you should always aim to keep to the foods in the 'eat this' column – such as brown rice and whole-wheat pasta – and these are the foods that are included in the suggested meal options. They are beneficial to both your overall health and weight-loss goals. For most of the carbohydrates and proteins, as well as fruit, portions are specified in the meal options in both the attack and lifestyle phases. Most vegetables (such as spinach and cucumber) can be eaten freely with your meals, and if portions are not specified, it means this is the case.

Anything with an asterisk denotes a healthy food (that is, an 'eat this' one) that need not be avoided but should be consumed in moderation due to its calorie content.

Fruit

EAT THIS	BE CAREFUL	STAY AWAY
All fresh fruit	Dried fruit with added sugar	Bananas
Dried fruit (no added sugar)*	Tinned fruit in sugar/syrup	Fruit cakes/crumbles
Tinned fruit in natural juices (no added sugar)		Fruit juice
		Fruit pies/pastries

Vegetables

EAT THIS	BE CAREFUL	STAY AWAY
All the following (fresh/ frozen/tinned in water)		
Artichokes	White potato	
Asparagus		
Aubergine		
Avocado*		
Bean sprouts		
Broccoli		
Brussels sprouts		
Butternut squash		
Cabbage		
Carrots		
Cauliflower		
Celeriac		
Celery		
Chives		
Corn		
Courgettes		
Cucumber		
Fennel		
Garlic		
Green beans		
Kale		
Leeks		
Lettuce (all varieties)		
Mangetout		
Mushrooms		
Onions		

EAT THIS	BE CAREFUL	STAY AWAY
Pak choi		
Parsley		
Parsnips		
Peppers		
Rocket		
Spinach		
Sweet potato		
Tomatoes		
Watercress		

Legumes

EAT THIS	BE CAREFUL	STAY AWAY
All the following (dried/ frozen/tinned in water)		
Black beans	Baked beans	
Broad beans		
Butter beans		
Cannellini beans		
Chickpeas		
Haricot beans		
Kidney beans		
Lentils		
Peas		

Fats and Oils

EAT THIS	BE CAREFUL	STAY AWAY
Avocado*	Butter	Full-fat mayonnaise
Coconut oil*	Groundnut oil	Hydrogenated vegetable oils
Flaxseed oil*	Low-fat mayonnaise	Margarine
Guacamole* (home-made)	Non-stick cooking sprays	Palm oil
Hummus* (home-made/ reduced fat)	Reduced fat margarine, trans-fat free	Shortening
Natural nut butters*	Sesame oil	Vegetable oil e.g. corn/ soya
Nuts (see Nuts and Seeds)*		
Olive oil*		
Olives*		
Rapeseed oil*		
Sunflower oil*		
Techina*		

Nuts and Seeds

EAT THIS	BE CAREFUL	STAY AWAY
Almonds*	Salted nuts	Caramelised nuts
Brazil nuts*		
Cashew nuts*		
Chia seeds		
Linseed/flaxseed		
Nut butters*		
Peanuts*		

EAT THIS	BE CAREFUL	STAY AWAY
Pecan nuts*		
Poppy seeds*		
Pumpkin seeds*		
Sesame seeds*		
Sunflower seeds*		
Walnuts*		

Grains and Carbohydrates

EAT THIS	BE CAREFUL	STAY AWAY
Barley	Air-popped/low-fat popcorn	Biscuits
Basmati rice	Fruit chutneys	Buttered popcorn
Brown rice	Honey	Cake
Brown rice cakes	Jam	Crisps
Bulgur	Low-fat (bought) bran/fruit muffins	Chocolate spread
Corn	Low-fat refined (white) crackers	Croissants
Dark chocolate*	Manuka honey	Doughnuts
Home-made healthy muffin/treat*	Maple syrup	French fries/chips
Kasha	Matza	Fried noodles
Oats, oatmeal, porridge, oatcakes	Molasses	Fried rice
Polenta	Muesli mixes	High-fat crackers (like Snackers)
Quinoa	Pretzels	High-fat granola
Rye	White bread, bagels, pitta	Milk chocolate
Rye bread	White pasta	Muffins (store bought)
Rye crackers	White rice (non-basmati)	Packaged waffles

EAT THIS	BE CAREFUL	STAY AWAY
Spelt	White tortilla wraps	Pastries
Sweet potatoes	Whole-grain breakfast cereals	Pies/pie crust
Wholemeal/multi-grain bread		Pizza
Whole-wheat bagels, pitta		Cereal bars
Whole-wheat couscous		Store-bought/bakery cakes
Whole-wheat low-fat crackers		Sweets (hard and jelly)
Whole-wheat pasta		Tarts
Wild rice		Refined high-sugar breakfast cereals
		Refined sugar (all varieties)

Proteins

EAT THIS	BE CAREFUL	STAY AWAY
Beans (see Legumes)	Chicken (dark), no skin	Bacon
Canned fish (all varieties, not in oil)	Duck (dark), no skin	Beef
Chicken breasts (no skin)	Feta cheese	Fried chicken
Edamame	Halloumi cheese	Fried fish
Eggs	Products made from lean chicken and turkey (like mince, burgers, meatballs)	Full-fat cream cheese
Fresh fish and shellfish (all varieties)	Turkey (dark), no skin	Lamb
Hummus*	Tinned fish (in oil)	Meat pies
Lentils		Offal (organ meats)
Low-fat milk and dairy products (see Dairy)		Pork
		Processed deli meats

EAT THIS	BE CAREFUL	STAY AWAY
Nut butters (see Nuts)*		Salami
Nuts (see Nuts)*		Sausage rolls
Smoked salmon		Sausages
Soya and soya products		Yellow/hard cheeses
Tofu		
Turkey breast; duck breast		
Veggie burgers (like Fry's brand, or home-made)		

Dairy Foods and Alternatives

EAT THIS	BE CAREFUL	STAY AWAY
Almond milk	Butter	Coffee creamers
Coconut water	Buttermilk	Condensed milk
Eggs	Coconut milk (full fat)	Cream
Egg whites	Fat-free/low-fat fruit yoghurt (with sugar)	Full-fat cream cheese
Fat-free/low-fat cottage cheese	Feta cheese	Full-fat yoghurt
Fat-free/low-fat cream cheese	Frozen yoghurt	Margarine
Fat-free/low-fat yoghurt (no sugar)	Halloumi cheese	Non-dairy cream substitutes
Oat milk	Light coconut milk	Whole milk
Rice milk	Reduced-fat processed cheeses	Yellow/hard cheeses
Ricotta cheese		
Skimmed milk powder		
Skimmed/semi-skimmed milk		
Soya milk (no added sugar)		

Beverages

DRINK THIS	BE CAREFUL	STAY AWAY
Bloody Mary*	Beer	Alcopops
Champagne*	Hot cocoa (low fat, low sugar)	Amaretto Sour
Coffee*	Pina colada	Cocktails mixed with energy drinks
Gin/vodka and diet tonic*	Rum and Diet Coke	Cocktails with cola mixers
Green tea	Vodka cranberry	Eggnog
Herbal tea		Energy drinks
Red wine*		Frozen daiquiri
Red/white wine spritzer*		Fruit juice with or without added sugar
Tea, regular		Hot chocolate (full fat and sugar)
Vodka and mineral water, with lemon/lime*		Malibu and Coke/fruit juice
Water, sparkling mineral water		Margarita
White wine*		Milky/creamy liqueurs
		Soft drinks, including diet sodas

Condiments and Sweeteners

EAT THIS	BE CAREFUL	STAY AWAY
All herbs and spices	Agave syrup, maple syrup	Chocolate spread
Chilli sauce (without oil)	Fruit chutneys	Full-fat bottled salad dressings
Stevia, xylitol	Hoisin sauce	Full-fat mayonnaise

EAT THIS	BE CAREFUL	STAY AWAY
Ketchup (reduced sugar and salt)	HP sauce	High-fructose corn syrup
Lemon juice	Jam	Refined sugar
Marmite	Low-fat mayonnaise	
Mustard	Molasses	
Salsa	Pure honey	
Soy sauce (reduced sodium)	Sweet chilli sauce	
Vinegars (all varieties)		

The fundamental principles of The Food Effect diet

These principles underpin The Food Effect diet, and following them will make losing weight achievable, as well as ensuring that maintaining a healthy weight will not be a lifetime struggle.

Eat whole, natural foods Avoid packaged, processed foods as much as possible. This means eating whole, natural foods that are close to, if not in, their natural state; for example, fresh fruit, vegetables, whole grains, nuts, eggs, dairy products and fish. The shorter the list of ingredients on a package of food, the better it is.

Make sure you never get too hungry Long gaps between meals disrupt your blood-sugar levels, leading to excessive hunger, cravings and stress eating. The outcome is that when you do eventually eat, you're so hungry that it takes a lot more food to feel satisfied, and it's unlikely that you'll binge on celery sticks. Eating small, healthy snacks between meals will help keep your blood sugar levels stable and your metabolism going strong. The suggested snacks in the meal options will guide you.

Stay well hydrated Often when we think we're hungry, we're actually just thirsty. Water aids weight loss by keeping your cells functioning at their fat-burning best, and also helps your kidneys to flush out excess toxins and chemicals, which may be slowing down your metabolism. Make sure you drink plenty of water throughout the day, as well as one to two glasses *before* every meal or snack you have. See more on this in The Food Effect rules (page 30).

Slow down your eating and enjoy your food Focus on the food you're eating and don't wolf it down. Avoid eating dinner in front of the TV or lunch in front of your computer; take time out to enjoy your meal and actually pay attention to what you're eating. This will ensure that your brain registers when you've eaten enough – before it's too late.

Eat healthy fats – don't go fat-free This means eating good, healthy unsaturated fats found in nuts, peanut butter, avocados, olive oil and various other healthy oils. Incorporating good fats into your diet will help reduce sugar cravings, increase energy levels and keep you fuller for longer. While too much fat can cause weight gain, too little of the *right* fats prevents your cells from functioning properly, which affects fat metabolism, hormone balance and energy – all leading to weight gain. There's more detailed information on fats in Chapter 6.

Don't shun carbs Instead, stick to whole-grain, unrefined carbohydrates such as oats, wholemeal or rye bread, brown rice, sweet potatoes and quinoa. Slow-release carbs from whole-grain sources will give you the get-up-and-go you need to stay active and full of energy, while keeping your metabolism going strong and steady all day (and night). They are also great sources of fibre and various other essential nutrients.

Know yourself and be realistic Each of us has different needs, goals and preferences, combined with different body types and genetic make-up. You have to recognise your individual needs and be realistic about the changes you can make. For example, if you enjoy having your evening snack late at night, there's no point trying to force yourself to eat it earlier in the day. Evidence has refuted the myth that calories eaten late at night are 'worse', and has proven that a calorie is a calorie is a calorie. Whether you eat it at 7 p.m. or midnight, there's no difference; it's your overall daily consumption that counts, which is why you're allowed an evening treat every night.

Eat a rainbow Whether they are fresh, frozen or tinned – try to increase and vary your intake of fruit and vegetables. You'll feel so much better and your body will benefit from all the added vitamins, nutrients, antioxidants and fibre. Diets rich in fruit and vegetables have been proven to decrease the risk of heart attacks, strokes and a variety of cancers, and healthy, glowing skin is another by-product of eating a colourful, varied diet.

Know your portions Just because it's healthy, it doesn't mean that it can't make you gain weight. Even if you stick to healthy foods, you still have to watch your portion sizes and quantities when consuming foods such as nuts, hummus, avocado, olive oil and dark chocolate (in other words, all the things marked with an asterisk in the tables). They may be healthy but that does not mean that you can eat them freely. There's definitely a benefit in consuming a little olive oil, but pouring it liberally over your pasta and dipping your bread in it will lead to excessive calories and weight gain. The same goes for nuts – learn what a normal serving size looks like (it's very easy to eat a whole big bag of nuts) and limit yourself to that.

The Food Effect rules

These rules go hand in hand with the above principles for healthy eating and weight loss. If you follow both sets of guidelines, you'll be guaranteed weight-loss success, and will look and feel better than ever. As I said earlier, The Food Effect diet is all about being the best version of you – so there are no excuses for not following these rules.

Prepare, prepare, prepare This is the golden rule of healthy eating habits. The more organised you are, the easier, and more likely, healthy eating and living will be. Make your own lunch if possible, pre-chop vegetables to have on hand for meals and snacks, and keep your fridge and cupboards stocked with the right healthy foods.

Avoid highly processed and packaged foods as much as possible Read the labels on food products – don't buy what you can't pronounce or have never heard of.

Don't go hungry Never go more than 3–4 hours without having something small to eat. Always carry your healthy snacks with you if you know you're going to be out and about for a while or working long hours. For convenience, all snacks are listed daily in your plan so there's really no excuse. But . . .

Don't graze Eating regularly does not mean that you should be constantly picking throughout the day. A few nuts here and there do add up. Stick to your three meals and two snacks per day – and nothing outside of that. Have them whenever you feel it suits you best to do so.

Ditch the white stuff Cutting out the white stuff is one of the easiest ways to lose weight and improve your health. Most processed, refined foods (think sugar, white bread, flour, pasta and sugary, low-fibre cereals – *not* egg whites, cauliflower and white fish) are just empty calories with little fibre and goodness.

Don't cut out all starchy foods As noted in Chapter 3, this would be a recipe for a long-term 'diet disaster'.

Eat good fats As explained in Chapter 6, you need some good fat in order to burn fat. This means eating good, healthy unsaturated fats found in nuts, peanut butter, avocados, olive oil and various other healthy oils. These are all included (in specified amounts) in the plan, as they are proven to lower the risk of heart disease and aid the body in the absorption of vitamins and minerals, as well as helping with satiety, cravings and weight loss.

Avoid trans-fats Often listed under the names 'hydrogenated oil' or 'hydrogenated vegetable fat', and found in many processed foods, these are toxic and have no health benefits whatsoever.

Eat vegetables and fruit You can eat as much salad, and fresh, steamed, stir-fried and baked vegetables as you like (within the specified meals), as long as they don't have added dressing or oil (apart from the amount specified in the plan). You can add as much lemon juice, balsamic vinegar or apple cider vinegar as you like. Fruit is also included in healthy, specified portions in the plan.

Eat slowly and chew thoroughly Take time to enjoy and savour all your food (meals and snacks). Chewing your food properly will aid efficient digestion, stop you from overeating and reduce any uncomfortable bloating you may experience from eating too quickly.

Drink plenty of water As well as keeping yourself hydrated throughout the day, make sure you drink 1–2 glasses of water before *every* meal or snack you have. If you have difficulty drinking enough plain water (around 2 litres a day), herbal teas, green tea (hot or iced) or lemon in hot water are all just as good.

No sugary soft drinks or fruit juice The reason for this is explained in Chapter 3.

Weigh yourself Weigh yourself first thing in the morning, after you've gone to the toilet, without any clothes on. In the attack phase I'll be advising you to weigh yourself every day for the first four weeks. The theory behind this, and why it is beneficial for weight loss, is explained in Chapter 11, which introduces you to phase one and starting the attack phase. After the first four weeks, once you're at the lifestyle phase, you should weigh yourself in the same way, once a week.

Start your morning with a mug of warm water and apple cider vinegar It's better than warm water and lemon – often promoted as the healthiest way to start the day – so my advice is to kick off the morning with a mug of warm water and apple cider vinegar. Put a tablespoon of apple cider vinegar – a wonder food with lots of healing properties – into a mug of warm water; drinking this will hydrate you and cleanse your digestive system. More effective than a probiotic, it's the perfect way to set up your body for its daily food intake ahead, as well as helping to prevent bloating. Even though it's a *vinegar* it actually neutralises acid, and puts your body in a good pH balance so that your internal systems work well. It can also kill bad bacteria in the stomach and intestine, and promotes good gut bacteria. I must admit that I personally struggle with the taste 'straight up' so I add a teaspoon or two of stevia to make it more palatable. There's absolutely no health downside to doing this, so do try it.

Have a big hot drink with your breakfast (and mid-morning) This provides a warm, comforting start to the day that, combined with a good breakfast, leaves you feeling satisfied for the day ahead. It can be tea, coffee, herbal or green tea. Stick to skimmed, soya or almond milk only, with no added sugar, but sweeteners such as stevia and xylitol are allowed with no restriction (see Chapter 3).

A word on caffeine While excess caffeine is obviously not good, caffeine from good-quality coffee (*without* added sugar, syrups or whipped cream) is packed full of antioxidants and has been shown to have tremendous health benefits. When consumed before a workout, it has also been shown to boost performance and stamina while exercising. Keep to a maximum of two coffees a day, preferably early in the day – not late afternoon or evening, so as not to disrupt your sleep.

Limit (but don't shun!) alcohol There are many health benefits to alcohol as long as it's consumed in moderation and you stick to the right choices. Drink no more than three glasses a week during attack phase, and a maximum of one per night (up to seven drinks a week) once on the lifestyle phase. Keep to the drinks listed under 'drink this' in the table (see page 27), although it's fine to drink those in the 'be careful' category occasionally. Sticking to this limit will help you lose weight, clear your head and improve your energy levels, without making you cut out alcohol completely. For more on alcohol, see Chapter 9.

Don't give up or get despondent We're all human and have our ups and downs. While you are aiming to be disciplined in your food choices, The Food Effect healthy-eating lifestyle is not intended to starve or deprive you. If you do slip up, it's certainly not the end of the world. Don't feel as though you've failed and then set yourself back further by going on a total binge fest – just accept it and move on.

Enjoy your Food Effect journey and remember that as long as you continue to be consistent in the process, you will reap the benefits and get fantastic results.

*

The more stringent rules specific to the attack phase (the first twenty-eight days) are laid out in Chapter 11. Both phases of The Food Effect diet (all meal and snack options) are based on the foods in the tables in this chapter, incorporating mainly 'eat this' foods, and avoiding anything from the 'stay away' list.

CHAPTER 3

Don't Shun Carbohydrates

Dispelling the myths

In today's dieting age, carbohydrates – or carbs as they're commonly known – are seen as the enemy – often associated with piling on the pounds and increasing body fat. In reality, nothing could be further from the truth. Carbohydrates can actually help you to reach your weight-loss goals – you just need to know which ones to eat, and which ones to avoid.

Almost everyone knows that a healthy diet is the key to losing weight, but for some reason the first thing people often think they need to do is stop eating carbs. In fact, cutting out carbs might lead to weight loss at first, but it won't be sustainable and you'll end up tired, lethargic, cranky and irritable. You will also pile on the pounds the minute you start eating 'normally' again – because living off dry tuna, chicken, lettuce leaves and steamed broccoli is not sustainable for the rest of your life.

The fact is that cutting out carbs can slow down your metabolism and the process of fat burning, preventing you from reaching your goal weight, because your body needs them to function properly (more on this later). Without carbs, your body will actually hold on to excess fat because it's lacking its main energy supply. Cutting out all starchy foods is therefore a major diet disaster; however, when eating them, you must stick to the right ones. These include whole-grain unrefined carbohydrates such as wholemeal or rye bread, quinoa, whole-wheat pasta, brown rice, sweet potatoes and oats (i.e. everything listed under the 'eat this' column for carbohydrates in the tables on page 24). These are great sources of fibre and full of a variety of other nutrients.

While it's widely accepted that highly processed refined carbohydrates (those listed under the 'stay away' column in the same table) are bad for health and can contribute to weight gain, whole-grain complex carbohydrates are actually full of fibre and various other essential nutrients, which help keep you full for longer by regulating your appetite – the key to successful sustainable weight loss.

Before getting on to practical aspects such as guiding you on portion sizes to enable you to lose weight without cutting out the carbs, here is some basic nutritional information to help you understand The Food Effect approach to carbohydrates.

What are carbohydrates?

Carbohydrates are our brain and bodies' main source of energy, which we all need to carry out everyday activities. Through my experience with countless clients, friends and family, as both a doctor and a nutritionist, I've seen the harm that cutting out carbs can do to people, in both the short and long term.

Insufficient carbohydrate consumption can cause the following problems.

Temporary unsustainable weight loss

When you reduce your carbohydrate intake, you may notice how quickly – as if by magic – the weight falls off. But it's not fat you're losing – it's water. When carbs are stored in the body in the form of glycogen, each gram of carbohydrate stores three to four times its weight in water. So as soon as you cut carbs and start using your glycogen stores, you'll lose a fair amount of water weight. This is particularly the case if you're on a high-protein diet that depletes your glycogen stores. While everyone loves seeing the numbers on the scales go down and this may give you a great boost, you will soon plateau once you've lost the extra water weight and your body clings on to its fat stores, as it's being depleted of its main energy source – carbohydrates. Once your body realises there's a food shortage, it goes into 'starvation mode' and your metabolism automatically begins to slow down in order to expend as little energy as possible. You will also be tired and irritable (as explained below), and as a result, will lose any motivation to stick to such unrealistic weight-loss plans. The outcome is that the weight loss will taper off and you will stop losing weight entirely. Moreover, when you do begin eating carbs again (because such plans are unsustainable in the long term), you will pile on the pounds *even more* than normal, as your whole metabolism and ability to burn carbs will have slowed down.

Muscle cramps and low energy levels

Anyone who carries out physical exercise will need to replenish glycogen stores that are depleted during exercise, making carbohydrate consumption essential – especially post-workout. Carbohydrates are the body's main source of energy for fueling all exercise, including cardio and resistance training. Cut out carbs and your energy levels will drop. The result of decreased levels of your body's stored carbohydrates (glycogen) is a decreased ability to produce power, and poorer workouts mean poorer results. Whole-grain carbohydrates are an important source of iron, magnesium and B vitamins, all of which are critical in maintaining energy levels and muscle function. Many people are already deficient in magnesium, so without a healthy supply of the right carbs, all of your cells slow down and your muscles suffer as a result.

Fatigue and poor mental function

Carbs are not only the body's main source of energy, but also the brain's. When you cut out carbs, the brain is essentially running on fumes – especially once glycogen levels are low and become depleted. Once all the glycogen is gone, your body breaks down fat and runs off carbon compounds called ketones. This results in a dry mouth, bad breath, weakness, tiredness, dizziness, nausea and 'brain fog' – you may even feel as though you have flu. Eventually, your body adapts to running on ketones so you get used to it, but you certainly won't be functioning at your best as this isn't the body's preferred fuel source. Carbohydrates also play a major role in maintaining hormone balance, which is vital for sufficient and optimal bodily function.

Cravings

If your blood-sugar levels are irregular (which can be a result of either insufficient carbohydrate consumption or eating the wrong carbs), you are more likely to crave 'bad' foods. The key is not to avoid carbs, but to make sure you consume the right ones. The tables in Chapter 2 are a good guide to which carbs will help you achieve your goals. Contrary to popular belief, carbohydrates are also what muscles want and need for optimum functioning – they are what refuels them. When we don't replenish our stores (by cutting them out when dieting, for example), our bodies produce hunger hormones to encourage us to seek them out. Our body will do whatever it takes to let us know it needs food. Hunger, deprivation and cravings are certainly not the best basis for weight-loss success.

Constipation

Whole-grain carbohydrate intake (what The Food Effect lifestyle promotes) is a major factor in how much fibre you consume. Fibre, found in whole grains, fruit and vegetables (see 'eat this' table on pages 20–22 and page 24), not only helps to stabilise blood-sugar levels, thereby preventing hunger and cravings, and reducing the risk of obesity and chronic diseases such as diabetes and bowel cancer, but it also helps to keep your bowel habits regular.

Moodiness

When you cut out healthy carbohydrates, fruit and whole grains, your mental health and happiness go right along with them. This is not solely because you're living off boiled chicken breast and steamed broccoli (who wouldn't get moody?), but because carbohydrates, including whole-grain unrefined carbs, increase the brain's level of the feel-good hormone serotonin.

Different types of carbohydrate

Carbohydrates can be divided into two main types: simple (sugars) and complex (starch and fibre). The difference between the two lies in their molecular structure – simple carbohydrates have a simple molecular structure and complex carbs have a more complex one. This affects how they're broken down and absorbed by our bodies.

Simple carbohydrates

Simple carbohydrates are made up of one to two sugar molecules and are broken down and digested very quickly due to their simple structure. Examples of foods containing these carbs are sweets, cakes, biscuits, sugary drinks and sodas, white bread and white rice. When consumed, these foods are rapidly converted into sugars, which are directly absorbed in the blood in the form of glucose, leading to rapidly elevated blood-sugar levels. The glucose provides instant energy, but if not burned or used up (which it rarely is, unless these foods are consumed right before a workout), they are converted to, and stored as, fat – leading to weight gain and potentially its associated health issues. It's for this reason that these foods are placed in the 'stay away' or, at best, 'be careful' categories in the tables in Chapter 2.

Complex carbohydrates

These are made up of longer chains of sugar molecules than simple carbs and take longer to break down, requiring more time for digestion. This slows down the breakdown process, and supplies us with sustained energy and increased satiety, for a longer period of time. Examples of complex carbohydrates are brown rice, sweet potatoes, rolled oats and wholemeal bread. Since these carbohydrates require more time for conversion, they are constantly used up by the body and are not immediately converted to, or stored as, fat (unless eaten in large amounts, which is why portion sizes are specified in the meal options).

The Glycaemic Index

The Glycaemic Index (GI) is a ranking of carbohydrates from 0 to 100, according to how quickly they raise blood-sugar levels after they are eaten. As discussed earlier, simple carbohydrates raise blood sugar rapidly and therefore have a high GI, whereas complex carbohydrates take longer to break down in the body and thus have a lower GI, indicating that they don't cause a spike in blood-sugar levels. For this reason, these are always preferable.

Low-GI carbs

Extremely nutritious due to the abundance of vitamins, minerals and fibre they contain, these are the carbohydrates that are included in the The Food Effect meal plan. Because fibre cannot be digested by the body, it slows down the digestion of the digestible carbs, so blood-sugar levels do not spike – thereby promoting satiety and helping to manage cravings. Low GI carbs (such as the complex carbohydrates mentioned above) give steady energy levels, which are extremely beneficial throughout the day, including after exercise.

Sweet potatoes, for example, have a lower GI than white potatoes, as they take longer to break down into sugar in the body. Sweet potatoes are therefore the healthier choice compared with white potatoes, and certainly a wiser option for people who have diabetes or are managing high blood-sugar levels. Additionally, sweet potatoes are richer in the antioxidant beta-carotene, which helps defend against cellular damage that can lead to cancer and heart disease. Thus you'll see a lot of sweet potatoes in The Food Effect meal options. Apart from being super healthy, they're super tasty, too – so you won't feel deprived of delicious carbs. You can enjoy them mashed or baked whole or in wedges. If you're not a sweet potato lover already, your taste buds will soon get used to them, as you replace your white spuds for them. You can add different herbs and spices to sweet potatoes, such as cinnamon and rosemary (sweet), or salt, paprika and chilli powder (spicy and savoury), to suit your preference.

A note on rice

While I advocate brown rice over refined white rice, white basmati rice is an exception. It is higher in protein and fibre than regular white rice, and is actually considered a whole grain, so you can enjoy it guilt-free, as long as you stick to the same portions specified for brown rice in all the meal options in both the attack and lifestyle phases. White basmati rice has a lower GI than regular white rice, meaning it is broken down more slowly, keeping your blood sugar levels stable, in a similar way to brown rice.

High-GI carbs

Foods with a high GI, such as those mentioned under simple carbohydrates (see page 39), are rapidly digested and absorbed by the body, resulting in a spike in blood-sugar levels. When digested, they provide a large amount of glucose, which is usually not used or burnt off soon after, and will most probably be stored as fat, leading to an increase in body fat. By following The Food Effect diet you will naturally be avoiding these 'bad' carbs. Better yet, by including the right carbs, the diet will help you to banish cravings for these unhealthy, weight-loss sabotaging carbs, so you'll lose weight and keep it off without even trying.

A high level of insulin, the hormone released in response to glucose in the body, is one of the main contributors to fat storage around the tummy area. Swapping high-GI, refined simple carbohydrates for low-GI, unprocessed complex carbs, helps keep your insulin balanced, making those extra pounds and inches around the waist melt away.

Bottom line: avoiding carbs is *not* a good idea no matter what your weight-loss goals are. The most important thing is to review what type of carbs you eat and how much – and The Food Effect tables and meal plans will guide you on this.

The Food Effect take on sugar

Unless you've been living under a rock, you'll know that sugar is nutrition enemy number one. You'll also know that sugar (or rather a lack of it), plays a key role in losing weight and getting rid of unwanted fat. But is a 'sugar detox' really necessary, and if so, how should you go about it? Here is The Food Effect way.

Cutting out refined white sugar in its 'raw', granulated state, as well as in all those highly processed sugary foods and soft drinks (see 'stay away' in the table relating to carbs on page 25), is certainly essential for losing weight, increasing energy levels, improving skin and mood, getting rid of cellulite and burning fat. Excluding the things that offer little nutritional value, such as fizzy drinks, is an essential first step in reducing your sugar intake. But is it necessary to cut out fresh fruit (or even dried fruit in specified portion sizes) as we're advised to do in some of the latest fad diets? The answer is no.

You'll see that all fresh fruit (apart from bananas) is included in the 'eat this' column of the table (see page 20), and even dried fruit is allowed, with portion sizes specified in the meal and snack options. This is because fresh (and dried) fruit provides a wealth of vitamins, minerals and nutrients, and does not have the addictive properties – along with its empty calories – of refined white sugar.

Why avoid bananas?

While bananas are very nutritious, they are higher in calories and carbohydrate than other fresh fruit. For example, 100 grams of raw apple contains 52 calories and 14 grams of carbohydrate, whereas 100 grams of banana provides 90 calories and 23 grams of carbohydrate. So if you're eating 150–200 grams of fruit, the calorie and carb count is going to be far higher if you include banana. I don't think it's practical to tell people to have half a banana for a snack – one apple, pear or orange for example is more practical and realistic. Cutting out bananas and sticking to other fresh fruit has helped so many of my clients, and with so many other nutrient-rich fruit to choose from you won't be missing out.

However, during the first twenty-eight days (the attack phase), the only fruits allowed are apples, oranges, pears, grapefruit and berries. These fruits have the lowest GI, and as this initial phase is designed to wean you off refined sugar and carbohydrates, this will help you really see the effects of reducing your sugar intake. You'll be amazed at the difference it makes to your waistline, mood and energy levels. Occasionally, even during the attack phase, a small portion of dried fruit (such as figs or raisins) is specified. Once you move on to the lifestyle phase, all types of fruit are allowed apart from bananas. There are also plenty of delicious, indulgent, yet completely healthy recipes, and suggestions for snacks and sweet treats once you get on to this phase (Chapters 11 and 12 provide more specific guidance).

Fighting off the temptation of delicious-looking desserts, sweets, biscuits, cakes and chocolate bars in virtually every restaurant, supermarket and newsagent is daunting enough, but even more so when you realise that our brains are actually wired to crave sweet things. This is because refined sugar causes the neurotransmitter dopamine to be released in the brain. Dopamine is associated with our bodies' reward mechanism, so your brain remembers the incentive and signals you to perform the act again. Not many people can stop at one biscuit, sweet or square of milk chocolate, but you very rarely hear of people going on an apple binge. While eating high-GI refined sugary carbs just perpetuates these cravings, fresh fruit does not. It satisfies your sweet tooth in a healthy way, helping to banish cravings and preventing a surge in insulin and dopamine, so conquering cravings and weight gain at the same time.

Sugar has also been found to mimic the effects of opiates in the body. Opiates are addictive chemicals that are used widely for pain management. When a person is addicted to opiates and tries to stop taking them, the body goes into withdrawal. Quitting sugar, especially if you currently consume a lot of it, can cause withdrawal in a similar way. The symptoms can include irritability, fatigue, mood swings, headaches, anger, anxiety and dizziness. Although you're cutting out refined sugary carbs on The Food Effect diet, there's no need to cut out healthy fruit and make the process even harder.

The Food Effect diet and way of eating is specifically designed to make things easy, manageable and enjoyable, unlike extreme sugar-detox diets that make you cut out fruit entirely, leaving you feeling tired, moody, zapped of energy, and too down to find inspiration and motivation to 'keep going' and stick to any plan. With the inclusion of fresh and dried fruit, and low-GI carbs, you may have one or two days of slight difficulty – at worst – when initially cutting out your favourite sweet treats. Over time, however, you'll find that you naturally say no to sugar on a regular basis because you feel better without it, and you won't even have to think about avoiding it.

It's important to note that refined sugar can also be hidden in deceptive 'healthy' foods, such as granola, sports drinks and protein bars. So even if you cut out your morning croissant or pastry, you may unknowingly fill up on sugar from a seemingly innocent-looking cereal bar or flapjack, which causes the exact same spike in insulin, and the same craving cascade, as a junk-filled milk-chocolate bar or milkshake. So (fresh fruit aside), it's wise to know where all your sugar intake is coming from. Check the label on packaged cereal, protein bars and snacks, and if 'sugar' is listed in the first three ingredients, avoid the product altogether.

Fruit smoothies and juices cause a completely different reaction in the body compared to eating fresh fruit. They can easily contain more sugar than you should consume at once, so if you drink too many of them you may be fighting off sugar cravings for an entire day. Fruit juice is basically sugared water with all the fibre from the fruit extracted, and very little vitamin and mineral content remaining. This is why fruit juice is not included in the The Food Effect plan, and is under the 'stay away' column in the tables.

So, now you know what you're up against, what can you do

about it? Fortunately, it's very easy to break the sugar-craving cycle on The Food Effect plan. Simply avoid all the foods in the 'stay away' column of the tables, and follow the suggested meal and snack options instead. You'll be off the sweet stuff and on to a better, healthier, slimmer you in no time.

Sweeteners – take the scare stories with a pinch of salt

While the inclusion of fruit and whole-grain carbs will help keep you satisfied during your weight-loss journey, some of us have a naturally sweet tooth that needs to be satisfied, and while you definitely won't be allowed to sprinkle sugar on your cereal, why should you have to go without enjoying the taste when there's a perfectly safe and calorie-free way to do so? Additionally, having a large mug of sweet coffee or herbal tea can go a long way in helping to beat sugar cravings.

While xylitol and stevia might sound like sci-fi villains that people automatically assume are unhealthy, they are actually perfectly safe, natural sugar substitutes, or 'sweeteners'. Fears about their potentially toxic effects, ranging from diabetes, cancer, strokes and seizures, to vomiting, high blood pressure and dizziness, have all been cited but none of these claims have actually been proven. The American Food and Drug Administration and the European Food Safety Authority say they're completely safe, and I'd similarly advise you to take the scare stories with a pinch of salt. Real sugar is *far* worse for your weight and health in so many respects, and that's definitely been proven.

Stevia (my preference) is completely natural, as it is derived from a herb, and tastes far sweeter than processed sugar, so the amount needed to create the same level of sweetness is dramatically lower. Even better, it contains virtually zero calories and no 'nasties', and doesn't spike blood-sugar levels at all – making it the best option all round.

So many of my clients are scared of sweeteners such as stevia, yet they spoon regular refined white sugar into their tea or coffee. This makes absolutely no sense – refined white sugar (sucrose), with its high calorie content and need for insulin to break it down, poses the real risk of weight gain, obesity and Type 2 diabetes. Sweeteners, on the other hand, have zero (or very few) calories, do not raise insulin levels and are approved as safe for diabetics. As these sweeteners are absorbed more slowly than sugar, they do not contribute to high blood-sugar levels or the resulting hyperglycaemia caused by insufficient insulin response. This characteristic has also proven beneficial for people suffering from metabolic syndrome (a common disorder in our Western society), which includes insulin resistance, hypertension, hypercholesterolemia and an increased risk of blood clots.

Interestingly, the sweetener xylitol is actively beneficial for dental health. It not only reduces cavities but numerous studies have shown that xylitol is effective in inducing remineralisation of deep layers of demineralised enamel in the teeth. This is because the perception of sweetness from consuming xylitol causes the secretion of saliva, which acts as a buffer against the acidic environment created by the microorganisms in dental plaque. The increase in salivation can return an acidic pH to a neutral range within a few minutes of xylitol consumption.

Interestingly, sufficient evidence has also found that xylitol (in chewing gum, lozenges, nasal spray and so on) reduces the incidence of acute middle-ear infection in healthy children.

While both the American Food and Drug Administration and the European Food Safety Authority approve the use of artificial sweeteners including aspartame (Equal) and saccharin (Sweet 'n Low), these are completely unnatural and made purely from artificial chemicals. I would advise sticking to only the natural sugar substitutes (that is, stevia and xylitol). These won't spike your blood sugar or affect energy levels, and will stop sugar cravings and aid weight loss.

You'll see that the addition of sweeteners such as stevia or xylitol (as well as all-natural ground cinnamon) is suggested in the meal options. You can rest assured that you'll be doing your health and weight a favour by cutting out refined white sugar and using these natural sweeteners instead.

Raw honey, agave nectar syrup and pure maple syrup are also natural sweeteners that will tingle your taste buds. They are included and allowed in moderation in The Food Effect plan. They're rich in calcium, iron, B vitamins and potassium, and are certainly better for you than the processed sugar you find in sweets and unhealthy baked goods. As they're higher in calories, however, their amounts are limited and specified (unlike for calorie-free stevia) in the meal options.

In short, if you have a sweet tooth and like your coffee, tea, porridge and yoghurts to taste sweet, go ahead and add some natural Food Effect-friendly sweetener. A bit of stevia is far better than sugar.

Wheat and gluten – a few more myths debunked

'Wheat makes you fat' and 'removing gluten from your diet will help you lose weight' are two popular nutrition myths you may have heard – but there is absolutely no medical or scientific basis for this to be the case for the average healthy individual.

The world of health and fitness is awash with misinformation. I see so many clients who have been exposed to repeated misinformation, and have gone 'gluten free' (and/or 'dairy free') for no real reason, with the result that they are then left with very restrictive diets and even a fear of certain foods, for *no real reason*. (I am not referring to those who have a genuine intolerance to certain foods or food groups, and might need to eliminate them accordingly.)

The myth that 'wheat makes you fat' is in part a result of the 'clean-eating' diet craze, which blames wheat for obesity and a host of other medical conditions, with people making unsubstantiated claims that cutting out gluten cured all their ailments. Yes, people who eat a lot of refined wheat flour in foods such as white bread, biscuits and pastries will indeed gain weight; and yes, if they cut out these refined foods and eat a more balanced diet (as you will be doing on The Food Effect diet) they'll lose weight. But it's not because of the wheat; it's because they've improved their overall diet and meal balance. There have been no scientific studies that support wheat as the culprit for our obesity epidemic, or that support a wheat-free diet for weight loss. The best thing you can do for weight loss is to replace refined white wheat (such as that in white bread, pastries, cakes and biscuits, made with refined white flour) with whole grains (like those found in wholemeal bread, or muffins made with wholemeal flour), to increase your fibre intake so that you'll feel fuller and avoid cravings.

In terms of gluten, increasing diagnoses of coeliac disease (a true gluten intolerance), due to heightened awareness and better screening, has put gluten in the spotlight in recent years. However, many people mistakenly think that a gluten-free diet is the key to weight loss. This couldn't be further from the truth. People are blaming gluten for symptoms when it's not the underlying cause. It's trendy and cool, and many celebrities are endorsing gluten-free diets, so people jump on the bandwagon. Going on a gluten-free diet can be unnecessarily expensive, and will not guarantee better health or weight loss. There is no evidence to suggest that weight or fitness is improved in any way when following a gluten-free diet.

In fact, a recent study in the *Journal of the American Medical Association* showed that the growing popularity of gluten-free diets, endorsed by high-profile celebrities, has been driven by fashion choices rather than diagnosed health problems. Researchers found that there has been no increase in the numbers of those suffering from coeliac disease in the past six years, yet those on a gluten-free diets have risen threefold. The authors say that other reasons are also clearly driving the trend, including a misinformed public perception that gluten-free diets are healthier, and people are increasingly self-diagnosing themselves with 'gluten sensitivity' without having the typical symptoms of coeliac disease. The study confirms that, unsurprisingly, the rising popularity of gluten-free diets is not accounted for by any increase in clinically proven cases of coeliac disease. The huge number of 'gluten-free foods' now available on supermarket shelves is also helping to boost the numbers of those shunning wheat. Sales of gluten-free products reached £184 million in the UK in 2015, up 15 per cent from the previous year, so savvy marketing also plays a huge role in influencing food choices.

Gluten-free diets are specifically designed for the 1 per cent of the population that does have coeliac disease and the 6 per cent with non-coeliac gluten sensitivity. For these people, foods containing gluten, such as wheat, rye and barley, can lead to a host of symptoms including gastrointestinal problems, skin rashes and anaemia. For the rest of the population, however, gluten should not pose a problem. Whole-grain wheat, barley and rye are nutritional powerhouses; they are good sources of fibre, B vitamins, vitamin E, iron, magnesium and antioxidants – all of which are essential for healthy living and disease prevention. Additionally, many gluten-free products are higher in calories and other unhealthy ingredients than their gluten-containing counterparts (as well as being much more expensive), but people are conned into thinking that anything with a 'gluten-free' label must be healthier and will help with weight loss, when this is nothing more than a myth.

The Food Effect diet is the last 'diet' you will ever need. As you can see, you will no longer be focusing on avoiding carbohydrates or gluten, as so many other diets will have you do. On The Food Effect diet, you'll be eating plenty of carbohydrates in order to start dropping pounds.

CHAPTER 4

The Food Effect Guide to Protein

More than just chicken and tuna

Before we get on to the numerous reasons to cut out or at least cut down on red meat in Chapter 5, I'll first share some basic facts on the science of protein.

What is protein?

If you were to ask most people what protein is, how the body uses it and what foods are good sources of it, most would answer that it's used to build muscles, and is found in meat, chicken and eggs. Now although none of that is inaccurate, it's just the tip of the iceberg. Proteins aren't solely required to help the body build muscle, and they certainly aren't only found in meat and eggs. They are required for virtually every bodily function. They are the primary building blocks of the body. Our muscles are made from protein, but so are our skin, hair, nails, eyes, bones and all our organs. Additionally, our hormones, enzymes and blood cells are mainly made up of proteins. Together with water, protein is the most abundant substance in the human body. So while I may not be telling you to tuck into a steak very often, I certainly think protein is essential and you definitely won't be skimping on it.

Eating plenty of protein throughout the day (along with whole grains, fruit, vegetables and healthy fats), will improve body composition, promote satiety, increase calorie burning and improve insulin control. All your meal and snack options in both phases of The Food Effect diet have been perfectly designed to do this.

Let's look at a few protein-containing foods that have been the subject of controversy and confusion.

Why The Food Effect diet does not exclude dairy foods

Due to the recent craze for low-carb diets and an increase in allergies, milk has got a bad reputation, but for no good reason. Cutting back on the amount of dairy foods you eat can actually signal the body to make more fat cells. When you don't have enough calcium, your body tries to hold on to whatever's there. This triggers the release of a compound called calcitriol, which, according to a study in the *American Journal of Clinical Nutrition,* increases the production of fat cells.

In some parts of the world, particularly in Africa and South Asia, where dairy farming is relatively new, lactose intolerance is widespread. However, in the West, dairy foods have been part of our diet for centuries and lactose intolerance is much less common. Owing to our long history of dairy farming, and therefore the availability of dairy foods, we tend to produce decent levels of lactase, the enzyme that helps us to digest lactose, so most of us in the West tolerate dairy products well.

Dairy is a hugely important food group, packed with protein, calcium, magnesium, phosphorus and fat-soluble vitamins and minerals, all essential for bone and dental health. Milk sugars (the afore-mentioned 'lactose') do not cause dental problems and are fine for the vast majority of us.

Research has shown that milk is better than water or sports drinks at helping the body to recover from exercise, because of all its abundant vitamins and minerals. For adults (and certainly children), it should be a key part of the daily diet.

Recommended daily intakes of dairy foods are slightly higher for adolescents than for any other age group due to their rapid bone growth, and because these are the years when bone structure is laid down for life. But this remains an important food group for everyone, right up to old age. Men and women over the age of nineteen need 700–1,000mg of calcium per day. A pint of semi-skimmed milk, for example, provides 693mg, and low-fat natural and Greek yoghurt are even richer sources of calcium than milk. You can also get calcium from other non-dairy sources such as almonds, sesame seeds, tahini and spinach. My advice is to aim for three portions of calcium-containing foods each day. These can include milk or yoghurt with breakfast, a yoghurt or a handful of almonds and fruit as a snack, a serving of cottage or feta cheese in a salad at lunch, and dark green leafy vegetables, such as spinach and broccoli, in the evening. That's all very manageable.

Although after the age of twenty-one we no longer build bone density, we can help to maintain it by keeping up our calcium intake. Consuming sufficient dairy foods can help to protect against osteoporosis in later life. Calcium also helps maintain muscle mass, which improves metabolism, helping you to burn calories more efficiently throughout the day.

Aside from being an excellent source of protein, calcium and phosphorus, all crucial for bone health, dairy products are a good source of fat-soluble vitamins, especially vitamins A and D. Low levels of vitamin D have been associated with increased fat storage, among many other health problems (see also page 127). Vitamin D deficiency also causes the brain to issue hunger-signalling hormones, tempting you to reach for the digestive biscuits and sugary milk chocolate. Additionally, calcium-rich diets have been found to aid weight loss, but vitamin D is required to regulate calcium absorption. So drinking milk is a real win-win.

And if you're worried about the sugar in milk, it is important to note that milk sugars (lactose), do not count towards the new recommended limits for *added* sugars of just 30g (6 teaspoons) per adult, per day.

For all these reasons you'll see plenty of dairy options (including Greek yoghurt, natural yoghurt, cottage cheese and other low-fat non-processed cheeses) in The Food Effect attack and lifestyle phase meal options. Yellow, hard processed cheeses are not allowed due to their high saturated fat and calorie content. If you genuinely suffer from lactose intolerance, soya milk, almond milk and other natural, dairy-free alternatives are all perfectly acceptable, too – just make sure they're fortified with calcium.

Full-fat, semi-skimmed or skimmed milk?

While the calorie and fat contents of full-fat and skimmed milk vary greatly (from 364 calories and 20g of fat per pint of full-fat milk, to only 199 calories and 0.6g of fat in skimmed milk), the difference in calcium content is negligible, with skimmed milk actually having *more* calcium and protein than whole milk. Calcium is present in the watery part of milk, and without the fat there is more protein and calcium in any given volume. As The Food Effect diet contains plenty of healthy fats (nuts, nut butters, avocado, oily fish and so on) you don't need the extra (saturated) fat and calories in full-fat milk. Ideally, stick to skimmed milk, but if you really can't get used to it, semi-skimmed milk is also allowed – but avoid full-fat milk and cream.

Debunking the myths about eggs

Eggs are another protein that you'll see featured in abundance in The Food Effect meal plans, be it for breakfast, lunch or dinner. Starting your day with eggs for breakfast has been shown to aid weight loss. They provide you with prolonged energy release, so you'll be less likely to opt for a sugary snack mid-morning. The same goes for eating eggs for lunch, and avoiding those notorious mid-afternoon sugar cravings.

When it comes to nutritious, 'weight-friendly' foods, the humble protein-laden egg is by far the most versatile and convenient, with a whopping 72.5 per cent pure protein and just 1.5g of fat. Despite this, there seems to be a lot of confusion, as well as dietary 'myths', surrounding the consumption of eggs – from the worry about eating them every day, to the common misconception that the yolks are 'bad for you'. This is certainly a topic I often get asked about. The 'egg debate' has been around for quite some time. Eggs used to be taboo because of their high cholesterol content – scientists had evidence that dietary cholesterol increased blood cholesterol, thereby increasing the risk of heart disease. But recent research has shown it's not quite as simple as that. Virtually all medical and nutritional experts now agree that eggs are absolutely fine to have regularly (as with all things, in moderation). In fact, a study in the *Journal of the American College of Nutrition* showed that people who ate eggs took in more essential nutrients (folate, vitamins A, E and B12) than those on an egg-free diet.

Cholesterol is an essential component of the body's cells and your body needs it to function. In fact, even if you don't consume any dietary cholesterol, your body will produce it anyway for essential bodily functions. Additionally, the research that initially linked eggs and heart disease has been shown to have many flaws, raising questions about the validity of the now outdated conclusion. One study actually found that the human body handles the cholesterol from eggs in a way that is least likely to harm the heart. Saturated and trans-fats are much greater dietary offenders when it comes to blood cholesterol. One whole egg (yolk included) contains only 1.5g of saturated fat and no trans-fats. All the latest medical research shows that the cholesterol in the yolks is actually the good, essential kind, not the bad kind that is responsible for raised cholesterol levels; there are therefore actually many more health benefits to be gained from eating eggs than avoiding them.

Eggs, as previously mentioned, are also a great source of protein, low in fat and carbs (they contain virtually none), and a fantastic source of folate, iron, zinc, selenium, vitamin D, B vitamins, choline and lutein. Choline helps to ensure proper functioning of the brain and combats inflammation, and lutein is a carotenoid (naturally occurring pigment) that is good for your eyes. B vitamins make eggs a great food for your hair and nails, and vitamin D boosts immunity, facilitates the absorption of calcium and phosphorus, and keeps your bones, teeth and muscles strong. Aside from the protein, all this nutritional goodness is packed into the yolk. In fact, the protein in egg whites is not as nutritious without the yolks (which themselves contain about 3g of hunger-busting protein). Also, when eaten on their own, egg whites aren't as satiating. The yolks balance out the amino-acid profile, so that the protein in the egg whites is more easily absorbed by our bodies. Abandon the yolk and you're likely to feel less satisfied, which can cause you to eat more later on. Egg yolks are also home to lots of essential but hard-to-get nutrients and antioxidants that have been shown to help prevent macular degeneration and cataracts. So to reap all the benefits, forget the 'egg white only' order, and enjoy the whole egg.

That being said, the majority of calories are in the yolk, so for weight-loss purposes, I would advise you to stick to a maximum of one whole egg (plus however many whites) per day (if you're eating eggs every day). So, for example, if you're making yourself scrambled eggs, an omelette or egg mayonnaise, use one whole egg plus two or three whites. If you only eat eggs a few times a week, two whole eggs at a time is fine.

In short, eggs are super-healthy. If you're looking to satisfy your hunger while packing in some good nutrition, eating eggs will definitely do the job. They are a wholesome, natural and inexpensive source of nutrients, and fabulously easy and fast to prepare. So, from now on, you can enjoy your eggs without the guilt.

A few more Food Effect protein favourites

There are other great, nutritious sources of protein, the benefits of which are outlined below.

Salmon

This is perhaps the ultimate nutritional superstar of fish. As well as being packed with protein, it's also an excellent source of potassium, selenium, vitamin B12, iron, niacin and phosphorus, and is one of the most beneficial to health because of its exceptionally high omega-3 fatty acid content. There's more about these healthy fats in Chapter 6, but among their array of health benefits, omega-3s aid weight loss by improving glucose sensitivity, reducing insulin resistance, reducing markers of inflammation, and speeding up fat oxidation. Eating salmon has also been shown to help protect against heart disease, Alzheimer's disease and many forms of cancer. In addition to helping to keep your heart ticking along nicely, the omega-3 fatty acids in salmon help to improve your ratio of lean muscle to fat, and give you gorgeous glowing skin. There are a number of options for incorporating salmon in The Food Effect meal plans and recipes.

Chicken

Lean chicken breast in particular is a great source of satiating protein that is extremely low in fat and incredibly versatile. It is also a very good source of niacin (important for energy production, fat, cholesterol and carbohydrate metabolism, and the production of sex and adrenal hormones), selenium (which helps prevent free-radical damage, thereby reducing the risk of cancers, cardiovascular disease, inflammatory diseases and premature ageing), vitamin B6 (critical in maintaining a healthy nervous system, red blood cells, hormonal balance and proper immune function) and phosphorus (essential for a wide range of bodily functions, including energy metabolism, DNA synthesis and calcium absorption).

Turkey

This is a good source of the amino acid leucine, which plays a role in blood-sugar levels and insulin function. By keeping your blood sugar levels steady, you are less likely to binge on other foods throughout the day. Turkey also contains another amino-acid called L-tryptophan, which releases serotonin (the calming, 'feel-good' hormone) in the body. Eating turkey has a soothing effect on the body and has been shown to help improve sleep. Choose the leanest white meat and eat it without the skin, to minimise unhealthy fat and calories.

Tuna

This fish is a fantastic source of satiating protein that is extremely low in fat and calories. It is also a very good source of potassium (important for heart health and lowering blood pressure), selenium and vitamin B12 (critical in DNA synthesis and maintaining a healthy nervous system). Tuna (along with other fish) has been shown to be beneficial for protecting against heart disease, Alzheimer's disease and many forms of cancer.

Greek yoghurt

This variety of yoghurt (including the fat-free version) is thicker and creamier than regular yoghurt, and provides a significant source of protein for a relatively small portion (a whopping 17g of protein in a small 170g container). Interestingly, 0 per cent plain Greek yoghurt provides the highest protein and calcium content of all yoghurt varieties. You'll see many options featuring Greek yoghurt (as well as natural yoghurt) in the meal plans. Delicious by itself or accompanied by fresh fruit and some agave syrup, Greek yoghurt is a wholesome and nutritious breakfast or post-workout snack. It is an excellent source of metabolism-boosting calcium (around 200–300mg per 170g container). It is also relatively low in lactose, making it easier to digest than other yoghurts for those who don't tolerate dairy products well. Aim for the lowest percentage of fat and skip the varieties with added fruit, toppings and sugars. Greek yoghurt is also a good source of probiotics, helping to keep your immune system and digestive tract healthy.

Cottage cheese

This cheese is another low-calorie, high-calcium, protein-packed option. Stick with low-fat cottage cheese. You'll see plenty of meal and snack options using cottage cheese in both savoury and sweet ways in The Food Effect meal plans for breakfast, lunch, supper and snacks.

Chickpeas

These pulses are a fantastic source of fibre and protein, and have a low GI. This powerful combination makes them particularly good at helping with weight management. In an Australian study, adults who ate 100g of chickpeas a day for four weeks ate fewer processed snack foods and felt fuller, compared to when they didn't include chickpeas in their daily diets. One 165g serving of cooked chickpeas provides 50 per cent of your daily fibre requirement, so it's no wonder that this legume provides long-lasting energy, keeps you feeling full, promotes good digestion, curbs appetite and has even been shown to help lower LDL (bad) cholesterol.

Lentils

Just 100 grams (raw weight) of these little legumes packs in 80 per cent of your daily requirement of fibre, which increases satiety and steadies blood-sugar levels. Lentils are also an excellent source of folate, which has been shown to be a key nutrient in preventing and treating depression, insomnia and muscular fatigue. Lentils are available in a variety of colours, and all pack a nutritional punch. Add them to salads, stews or a delicious vegetarian chilli, or try the recipe for Easiest Ever Red Lentil Soup (see page 227). Lentils are heavenly, healthy, hearty and filling.

Quinoa

Quinoa is one of the few vegetarian foods that is a complete protein, meaning that it contains all nine essential amino acids. It's also a rich source of fibre, magnesium, folate, copper, thiamin and vitamin B6. It is included in plenty of the meal options and recipes in The Food Effect plans.

Peanut butter

One serving of this tasty spread contains 5g of healthy mono-unsaturated fatty acids, which research shows can help keep you slimmer and keep belly fat at bay (see more on fats and the health benefits of nuts in Chapter 6). Almond and cashew butters are equally healthy, delicious alternatives. A 2-tablespoon serving of nut butter contains about 7g of protein, not to mention a host of vitamins, minerals and heart-healthy fats. Spread your choice of nut butter on cut-up fresh fruit (such as apple slices) or vegetables, or on whole-grain crackers, and you've got yourself a delicious, satisfying snack in minutes.

Pumpkin seeds

Next time you're craving something crunchy, instead of unhealthy crisps, grab some dry-roasted pumpkin seeds. A generous 28g serving packs in 8g of belly-filling protein, plus each little seed is a great source of fibre, vitamins, minerals, heart-healthy fats and antioxidants.

*

As you can see, The Food Effect diet encourages you to eat from a wide variety of healthy proteins, while reducing protein sources that arc high in saturated fat (more on this in the next chapter), such as fatty meats and full-fat dairy foods. Many people think that 'lean protein' means just chicken or fish – but hopefully this chapter has shown you that you can meet your protein requirements from a wide range of sources, and there is no need to believe the myths that eggs are 'bad for you' or that everyone should go 'dairy-free'.

With The Food Effect diet, you'll be relying on the healthiest protein choices, which reduce saturated fat in your diet (see Chapter 6 for more detail on specific fats), thereby promoting weight loss and keeping you full, slim and satisfied.

CHAPTER 5

Cutting Out Red Meat

The key to health, longevity and weight loss

You've read the good news in Chapters 3 and 4 – following The Food Effect diet won't mean you have to cut out carbs, gluten, fruit, poultry, fish, eggs or dairy foods (or healthy fats, as you'll read in Chapter 6). You'll be eating plenty of whole-grain carbs, fruit and vegetables, and an array of lean proteins, plant-based proteins and good healthy fats. However, you will be cutting out all red meat (that is, lamb, beef, pork and offal) during the attack phase (and limiting it to once a week once you get on to The Food Effect lifestyle). This may seem drastic if you 'live for' your red meat, but I'm by no means telling you to go vegan or vegetarian (as so many of the latest health fads and diets out there will do); you won't be living off beans and flaxseeds. You'll be allowed plenty of chicken, turkey, fish, eggs and dairy foods, and endless plant-based sources of protein; so it really is very achievable.

I've seen countless meat-loving clients, who have looked at me as if they thought I was either crazy or joking when I told them that they would be cutting out red meat once they start their Food Effect plan. They told me there was no way they could do it. I sympathised with their reaction, as I grew up in a South African home, a culture that 'lives for' its meat, so I made sure

I gave them plenty of alternatives, just as I have here, in The Food Effect meal plans and recipes. And guess what? After a few weeks they came back having lost weight, telling me they'd never felt better, and that they weren't even tempted by the red meat options in restaurants or at dinners served at friends' homes.

I had one South African male client who loved his red meat so much when I first met him, that he simply couldn't envisage cutting it out. But he did, lost weight, looked and felt amazing, and did so well on The Food Effect lifestyle that he never went back. During the time he was coming to me, he sent me a text message on his birthday saying that his wife was taking him to one of the finest meat restaurants in London, famed for its steaks, as a special birthday treat. He asked what he should do, and I replied that he should have a steak and enjoy it. When I saw him a week later at our follow-up appointment, he'd lost more weight and was continuing to do amazingly well. I asked him how his steak had been, and he told me, 'Before I came to you, I couldn't fathom cutting out red meat, and we went there and you even told me to enjoy a steak, but when we were ordering I didn't even want it and went for the chicken instead!' He said, 'I feel too good eating this way to go back to the red meat.'

Obviously, when I advise cutting out red meat, I don't envisage that it's something you should *never* have again, if you enjoy it. I'm all about balance and enjoying the odd indulgence every now and then. But the story above illustrates that even the biggest meat lovers can change their eating habits, and, trust me, once you do it, you won't regret it. What you gain is so much more than what you give up.

More than just meat-free Monday

Many people have been making the argument that our population has grown fat because we eat too much starch and sugar, and not enough meat, butter and fat. Recently the news has been full of articles citing research that saturated fat does not cause heart disease, as was once believed. The predictable headlines followed: 'Eat Bacon and Butter'.

But, alas, I have to tell you that bacon and red meat are anything but health foods. They might not be proven to *directly* cause heart disease but there is certainly enough conclusive evidence that they cause many other diseases, and they do nothing to help with weight loss. Moreover, obesity certainly *does* cause an endless list of health risks, including heart disease, diabetes, stroke, cancer and more. As mentioned earlier, I've seen the positive effects cutting out red meat has had on hundreds of clients, and now I'd like to share that information with you, too. Not only does eating red meat make you gain weight, it also affects your overall appearance.

Eating large quantities of red meat on a regular basis can seriously affect your skin and body's ageing process, as it has been shown to be particularly inflammatory for the skin. White meat such as chicken and turkey do not have the same effects. So both to improve your health and help you to keep the weight down, I advise swapping all red meat for leaner, whiter cuts, such as chicken and turkey breasts, during the Food Effect attack phase. Red meat can be reintroduced during The Food Effect lifestyle phase, but should still be saved for special (infrequent) occasions.

Your meal options are laid out in the two Food Effect phases in Chapters 11 and 12, but to summarise here – The Food Effect attack phase is completely red meat free (no lamb, beef or pork), but chicken and turkey are included, and The Food Effect lifestyle phase allows red meat no more than once a week (again, chicken and fish are freely included). If you're a meat lover, this may be hard news to bear, but as you'll read below, by cutting out red meat you'll be doing your health and weight a great favour. You may love nothing more than that juicy red steak or beef meatballs in sauce, but red meat is anything but favourable to your overall health and disease risk.

Nearly a third of people reduced their meat consumption during 2016, according to figures from the British Social Attitudes survey, as they tried to heed health warnings about processed foods such as bacon, ham and sausages. Forty-four per cent have cut back, plan to do so or are vegetarian already. Experts say that consumption is likely to fall further after the World Health Organization classified bacon, sausages and processed meats as 'group 1 carcinogens' – in the same category as alcohol and cigarettes – and ranked red meat, including beef and pork, as the next level down, 'probably carcinogenic'. The NHS says that too much red meat and processed meat can increase the likelihood of bowel cancer, with just two rashers a day raising the risk by a whopping 18 per cent.

Along with this very valid reason for cutting down on meat consumption for health reasons, as well as the benefits of it being more economical (the price of beef rose by 35 per cent in 2007–2014, and lamb increased 42 per cent in price), The Food Effect lifestyle phase advises cutting out red meat for weight loss, too.

When I first founded my nutrition practice and started seeing clients, my advice to cut out red meat was primarily driven by concerns about health and what I viewed as clear evidence that doing so was beneficial for health (blood pressure, cholesterol, cancer and heart-disease risk), despite what others out there were promoting. I placed all red meat in the 'stay away' column in The Food Effect tables (see page 25), and advised replacing red meat with chicken, turkey, eggs, fish and low-fat dairy foods, as well as pulses and other plant-based sources of protein. As a result, clients returned with improved blood results, lowered cholesterol and blood pressure, but also staggering weight loss – and they looked and felt so much better too.

The problem with red meat

The average Briton consumes 70g of red meat per day, with one in three of us consuming more than 100g per day. The World Health Organization warns that eating just 50g of processed meat per day (less than half a burger or half a hot dog) increases the risk of bowel cancer by 18 per cent. It also warns that evidence shows that eating 100g of fresh red meat per day is associated with a 17 per cent increased risk of cancer.

A compound called haem, part of haemoglobin (found in the blood), is what gives red meat its colour. It may, however, also damage the lining of the bowel. This is because it's broken down in the gut by a family of chemicals called N-nitroso compounds, which have been found to damage the cells that line the bowel, causing other cells to have to replicate more in order to heal. This increases the chance of errors developing in the cells' DNA, which is the first step towards cancers developing and increases the risk of cancer greatly.

Medical research has found clear links between the consumption of red meat and the development of colorectal, pancreatic and prostate cancers. Other chemical constituents that occur naturally in red meat include nitrates and nitrites. Once ingested, they can be converted to cancer-causing compounds. That's why processed meat (such as bacon, sausages, hot dogs, ham, salami and pepperoni) are even worse – the troublesome nitrates and nitrites present in fresh red meat are added in significant quantities to these meats as a preservative.

Red meat and disease risk

I've seen first-hand that people whose diets are high in red meat have significantly higher health risks, not just of cancer, but also of heart disease, high blood pressure, diabetes and many other chronic diseases (such as gout). Heavy meat consumption has also been linked to depression, loss of mental concentration and dementia. Heavy consumption of saturated fat (which is highest in red meat among all proteins) and trans-fat (a complete no-no on The Food Effect diet) can as much as double the risk of Alzheimer's disease. Meat is also one of the biggest factors behind the obesity epidemic, as it is closely correlated with weight gain.

According to the American Agriculture Department, Americans consumed 41 per cent more meat in 2000 than they did in 1950, and unsurprisingly, they're fatter and unhealthier than ever.

Research shows that animal protein, specifically in the form of red meat, may significantly increase the risk of premature mortality from all causes, including cancer, cardiovascular disease and Type 2 diabetes.

A study published in March 2014 found a 75 per cent increase in premature deaths from all causes, and a 400 per cent increase in deaths from cancer and Type 2 diabetes, among heavy consumers of animal protein who were under the age of sixty-five. Conversely, people who eat less meat and more fish have lower rates of breast, prostate and colorectal cancer. The Japanese, who eat a diet rich in fish and low in red meat, have one of the lowest rates of breast cancer in the world. Women who eat more red meat have also been shown to have a greater risk of breast cancer, with an increased risk of 22 per cent among those who eat red and/or processed meat.

More convincing evidence is presented in Dan Buettner's bestselling book, *The Blue Zones*. People living in areas of the world identified as having the highest concentration of centenarians in the world (the so-called 'Blue Zones') live on a predominantly plant-based diet. Such populations include the Sardinians, for example, who eat meat around once a week, and the people of Okinawa, Japan, who get only 7 per cent of their calories from protein (the majority comes from sweet potatoes).

High red meat consumption has also been shown to increase the risk of colorectal cancer in both men and women. The mechanism is most likely due to an altered microbiome, the collection of microbes that live in your gut and play a key role in your risk of diseases such as cancer, obesity and diabetes.

As mentioned, high red meat intake is also associated with being overweight, and being overweight is a known risk factor for several cancers, including bowel, breast and kidney cancers. While red meat might be high in protein, iron and zinc, it is devoid of fibre and other nutrients (found in abundance in plant-based proteins) that have a protective effect against cancer. Studies have also shown that people who eat a lot of red meat tend to eat fewer plant-based foods, which are protective against cancer.

Animal protein, especially in the form of red meat, also increases IGF-1, an insulin-like growth hormone that causes chronic inflammation, an underlying factor in many chronic diseases. Red meat is additionally high in Neu5Gc, a tumour-forming sugar that is linked to chronic inflammation and an increased risk of cancer.

Even the act of cooking red meat may increase your risk of cancer. When you grill or pan-fry meat, it can release heterocyclic amines and polycyclic aromatic hydrocarbons, substances that are known to cause cancer in animals.

Low-carbohydrate, high animal-protein diets, which so many people are foolishly advocating these days, promote heart disease via mechanisms other than just their effects on cholesterol levels. So even if saturated fat apparently doesn't *directly* cause increased blood cholesterol levels, it doesn't mean that it doesn't indirectly cause heart disease via other mechanisms. Arterial blockages may be caused by animal protein-induced increases in free fatty acids and insulin levels, and decreased production of endothelial progenitor cells, which help keep arteries clean and healthy. Red meat appears to significantly increase the risk of coronary heart disease and cancer due to increased production of a compound called trimethylamine N-oxide (TMAO), a metabolite of meat linked to clogging of the arteries.

Dr Garth Davis, a leading bariatric (weight-loss) surgeon, head of a thriving weight-loss practice in the USA and author of *Proteinaholic*, says meat consumption, *not* carbohydrates, is a chief cause of obesity and diabetes in our society. The EPIC (European Prospective Investigation into Cancer and Nutrition) study, which followed 512,000 people in ten countries for twelve years, concluded that meat, especially processed meat, is significantly associated with the development of Type

2 diabetes, while fruit and vegetable consumption is associated with a decrease in diabetes development. This is just one such example. Study after study has shown that people eating fruit and vegetables, and especially grains, exhibit remarkably low levels of inflammation, and have considerably lower levels of diabetes than the general population. There is also a great deal of research showing that the more animal protein and saturated fat people eat, the more at risk they are of developing high blood pressure, and that meat eaters suffer more heart disease. Dr Davis quotes a study by the University of Copenhagen that implicated saturated fat (highest in red meat) as having 'a causative role' in heart disease.

Meat consumption also increases oestrogen levels, causing an adverse 'oestrogen dominance'. Women who eat more red meat, and less fish and vegetables, have been shown to be more at risk of developing endometriosis, a chronic condition in which tissue that normally grows inside the uterus, grows outside it, often leading to severe pelvic pain and problems with fertility. As mentioned, high meat consumption is also associated with less fibre consumption, which serves to raise bad oestrogens and encourage the growth of harmful bacteria in your microbiome.

In addition, eating red meat increases uric acid and creatinine levels, thereby increasing your risk of kidney problems and gout. It also increases levels of hs-CRP, a marker of inflammation, and GGT, a marker of liver damage, so cutting it out will do your liver the world of good.

In case all that isn't enough to put you off, meat can be contaminated with superbugs, which can easily cause food-borne illness. In fact, 55 per cent of ground beef sampled by the Environment Working Group has been found to be contaminated. Cooking reduces, but does not eliminate, the potential for exposure to disease-growth promoters in ground beef. And while you may have heard that 'grass fed is better', it's still not great. Data is still lacking to show that grass-fed meat is better for your risk of cancer, oestrogen levels and weight gain.

Moreover, a recent 2016 scientific study has found that cutting down on red meat can lead to a longer life and prevent early death. The research indicated that a 3 per cent increase in calories from plant proteins – found in vegetables, pulses, grains, nuts and seeds – can reduce the risk of premature death by 10 per cent. The results added further evidence that the consumption of red and processed meats was linked to higher mortality. The study of 130,000 people found that the risk of death from heart disease fell by 12 per cent if there was a 3 per cent increase in the amount of plant proteins in the diet. In those who smoked, drank at least 14g of alcohol per day or were overweight, this risk was reduced even further. Replacing processed red meat with plant protein was linked to a 34 per cent lower risk of death from all causes for every 3 percentage points of calorie intake.

Dr Mingyang Song, the lead researcher from Massachusetts General Hospital in the US, said, 'Our findings suggest that people should consider eating more plant proteins than animal proteins, and when they do choose among sources of animal protein, fish and chicken are probably better choices.' This is exactly the way I suggest you should eat on The Food Effect programme.

Cutting out red meat – a key to healthy weight loss

Countless studies have shown that most men and women lose weight when they switch to eating more fish instead of red meat. One study that followed 1,730 male employees for seven years found that the more animal protein and saturated fats people ate, the more at risk they were of becoming overweight or obese. Given that around 65 per cent of British adults are overweight or obese, reducing intake of energy-dense fatty meats seems sensible. Too much animal protein, specifically in the form of red meat, can also cause inflammation and bloating, which no amount of crunches will get rid of. Meat is also extremely difficult to digest and disrupts intestinal bacteria, which leads to weight gain. In addition, most meat contains antibiotics, which can compound weight gain.

Some 'experts' may advocate low-carb, high-protein diets, but the science shows that this is completely the wrong way to be healthy. You might lose weight in the short term, but I assure you, you will put it all back on.

Scientific studies aside, this is something I've witnessed myself among all my clients who used to eat red meat regularly – they all lose weight once they cut it out and switch to lean poultry, fish, eggs and plant-based proteins, even if they are eating more carbo-hydrates than they were previously. This is my first-hand evidence in favour of The Food Effect lifestyle and approach. Not only do my initial 'meat and potatoes' clients come to me out of shape and overweight but they feel tired and sluggish, have stomach and digestive problems of all sorts, and lack the energy necessary to live an active, fulfilling life. Once they adopt The Food Effect approach to eating, and cut out (or even reduce) red meat con-sumption, they tell me they've 'never felt more alive', and they're no longer even tempted by a big fat juicy steak or burger – just like the client I told you about at the start of this chapter.

So, to reiterate, an optimal diet for preventing disease, as well as losing weight, staying slim and looking and feeling better, is a minimally processed, wholefoods-based diet that is low in red meat, harmful fats, and refined carbohydrates and sugar, and rich in fruit, vegetables, lean protein (those specified in the pre-vious chapter), whole grains, pulses, legumes and healthy fats, including oily fish, olive oil, nuts, seeds and avocados.

In case you're wondering how you will get enough protein and iron if you don't eat meat, just consider that the world's strongest primate, the gorilla, consumes enough of these nutrients by just eating fruit and vegetables and leaves (many green vegetables comprise 20–45 per cent protein), and unlike the gorilla, you'll be allowed to eat chicken, fish, eggs, dairy foods and plenty of plant-based sources of protein (nuts, beans, legumes and so on), so you definitely have nothing to worry about.

While you won't have to do any of the maths, as all your meal options are very clearly laid out in the twenty-eight-day Food Effect attack phase and in the lifestyle phase, here's some information on how it's possible to meet your protein requirements without consuming red meat.

Meat alternatives high in protein

Food	Protein amount
75g cooked lentils	18g protein
75g cooked split peas	16g protein
2 eggs	12g protein
250g 0% Greek yoghurt	23g protein
100g uncooked oats	7g protein
1 sweet potato	4g protein
40g chia seeds	12g protein
25g protein powder	20–25g protein
4 tbsp sunflower seeds	8g protein

In essence, it's virtually impossible to become protein deficient on a well-balanced, plant-based diet; and with the inclusion of chicken, fish, eggs and dairy foods, it's certainly impossible.

As Michael Pollan famously said: 'Eat food, not too much, mainly plants.' It seems there is enough good research to support this, too. As you work through The Food Effect programme, you can rest assured it's designed not just to keep you slim, but also to optimise health and prevent disease.

Reducing your red meat intake and following the options in both phases of The Food Effect diet will not only ensure that you lose the weight you've always wanted to lose and keep it off, but, if you are one of the many people facing a lifetime on medication for what are termed 'lifestyle diseases', it can reduce the need for these, thereby transforming your life.

CHAPTER 6

The Facts about Fats

Don't go fat-free – choose healthy fats

Entire books and countless studies have been written about dietary fats, but while you definitely don't need to know all the intricacies about fats to eat healthily, lose weight, stay slim and look and feel your best, there definitely are some basics that are worth knowing.

Good fats should not be feared

As described in Chapter 2, one of my top tips for healthy eating and weight loss is to eat healthy fats and not try go fat-free. You need some good fat to burn fat. This means eating healthy unsaturated fats of the type found in nuts, peanut butter, avocados, olive oil and various other healthy oils. These are included (in specified amounts) in The Food Effect diet, as they are proven to lower the risk of heart disease and aid the body in the absorption of vitamins and minerals. Incorporating good fats into your diet helps to reduce sugar cravings, increase energy levels and keep you fuller for longer. While too much fat can cause weight gain, too little of the right fats prevents your cells from functioning properly, which affects fat metabolism, hormone balance and energy – all leading to weight gain. That's why 'eat good fats' is one of The Food Effect rules, and 'avoid trans-fats' is another. Trans-fats are often listed under the names 'hydrogenated' or 'partially hydrogenated' vegetable oil or 'vegetable shortening', and are found in many processed foods. They are toxic and have no health benefits whatsoever (more on them later in this chapter).

Fats are a great source of energy and provide vital nutrients for the body. Additionally, they help the body absorb nutrients, such as vitamins and minerals from vegetables and salads, more efficiently. Some nutrients, such as vitamins A, D, E and K, and carotenoids (antioxidants found in many fruit and vegetables), require some dietary fat for absorption. That's why The Food Effect meal options always have some healthy fat included in them – whether it be in the form of avocado, a little olive oil, nuts, seeds or hummus. They're all designed to maximise the nutrition in your meal, without racking up the calories. However, even with all their health benefits, fats are the most calorie dense of all the macronutrients (containing 9 calories per gram, compared to 4 calories per gram for carbohydrates and protein), so you do have to be mindful of your portion sizes. Just because they're healthy, it doesn't mean that you can eat them freely, or that they can't make you gain weight. Even if you stick to consuming only healthy fats, you still have to watch your portion sizes and quantities when consuming foods such as nuts, hummus, tahini, avocado and olive oil (that is, all the things marked with an asterisk in the tables on page 23). There's definitely benefit in consuming a little olive oil, but as mentioned previously, consuming it in excess will lead to the consumption of too many calories and weight gain. The same goes for nuts – learn what a normal serving size looks like (based on the portions specified in the meal plans) and limit yourself to that.

Luckily for you, there's no guesswork involved. Whether it's avocados, nuts, peanut butter or even seeds on your porridge, I've done all the hard work for you and as long as you stick to my suggestions, you'll always be consuming exactly the right amount of fat to provide you with the optimum health benefits, without compromising your weight-loss goals.

Fats: the basics

The four main types of fat found in foods are saturated fats, monounsaturated fats, polyunsaturated fats and trans-fats.

Saturated fats, of which there are several types, are typified by the white fat you see marbled through red meat, or on the underside of poultry skin. It's fine to consume small amounts of saturated fat (such as a little butter), but excess amounts can encourage raised cholesterol levels. Coconut oil is an exception to this rule, due to its unique molecular structure. It can help the body burn fat and lower cholesterol (more on this below). In general, The Food Effect diet avoids large quantities of saturated fats.

Unsaturated fats (monounsaturated and polyunsaturated) are generally what I am referring to when I talk about 'healthy fats'. Foods that fall into this category include avocados, nuts, nut butters, oily fish such as salmon and mackerel, and olive oil. These are loaded with nutrients and have been shown to help with weight loss, keep you satiated and give you glowing skin. Omega-3 fats are the best known of this group of beneficial fats, and are found mainly in oily fish such as salmon, mackerel and herring; walnuts and linseeds (AKA flaxseeds). On top of their endless health benefits, omega-3s have been found to increase a hormone called leptin, which helps to promote satiety and banish unnecessary cravings. So embrace those omegas.

Trans-fats, which are completely artificial and manufactured, are what we really need to watch out for and avoid at all costs, as I've said above. These fats are usually created in a laboratory and are solid at room temperature. They are therefore useful to the food industry and are also popular with fast-food restaurants as they are cheap and long lasting. They are found in things like margarine, cakes, biscuits, pastries and fast foods such as chips. They've been linked to cancer, heart disease and diabetes, over and above weight gain and obesity. They've been shown to raise (bad) LDL cholesterol, and lower (good) HDL cholesterol, as well as blocking the absorption of good fats. It's for these reasons that foods containing these fats are listed in the 'stay away' column in the tables (see page 23). They do nothing to benefit your health, weight or well-being. Avoid them altogether.

Specific fats

Here is some essential information on the benefits and uses of specific fats.

Coconut oil

Coconut has an endless array of health properties that have been shown to benefit the heart, brain and digestive system due to its unique healthy fat content, antibacterial effects and balance of dietary fibre, protein, antioxidants, vitamins and minerals. The rich source of healthy fats – medium-chain triglycerides (MCTs) – found in coconut flesh and oil, has been shown to help lower the risk of heart disease by increasing healthy (HDL) cholesterol without raising unhealthy (LDL) cholesterol. These wondrous MCTs also help with weight management, by reducing appetite, boosting metabolism and increasing the activity of fat-burning cells.

Coconut oil is brilliant for cooking due to its high smoke point. This means that it is more stable, and less easily damaged and chemically altered when heated to high temperatures, compared with other oils, such as extra-virgin olive oil. The latter is super healthy, but is better for drizzling and dressings than heating and cooking. Although coconut oil is a saturated fat, it's a unique kind, and one I'm in favour of (unlike the saturated fat found in red meat and full-fat dairy foods, such as hard yellow cheeses), and it is allowed in moderation on The Food Effect diet.

Extra-virgin olive oil

This contains more healthy monounsaturated fatty acids than any other natural oil, plus a small amount of iron and a good level of vitamin E, a super-antioxidant. One compound found in olive oil, oleocanthal, is an anti-inflammatory. The downside of extra-virgin olive oil is that it has a relatively low smoking point, so that its flavour and some of its nutritious properties start to degrade at high heats. It's best used in dressings and on salads. However, light refined olive oil (not extra virgin) is safe to heat and use for roasting, cooking and frying. It possesses many of the same health benefits as extra-virgin olive oil.

Sesame oil

This oil has far fewer minerals and vitamins E and K than olive oil, but it does have good polyunsaturated fat levels, so it provides some healthy omega-3 fatty acids. It has a smoking point similar to that of coconut oil, and can be heated to 200°C without any negative effect. It has a bold flavour that best compliments Asian and stir-fry dishes. Use sesame oil sparingly due to its rich flavour and high calorie count.

Butter

You'll notice that butter is in the 'be careful' column in the tables (see page 23). This is because it's definitely not as bad for health as completely unnatural, highly processed margarine (in the 'stay away' column), but it certainly doesn't match up to the health benefits of the 'eat this' healthy fats, such as olive oil, nut oils, nut butters, hummus, tahini and avocado. It is therefore not actively encouraged on The Food Effect diet (and certainly not allowed during the attack phase), but it is preferred over margarine as a spread, or to cook and bake with once you are living The Food Effect lifestyle. It can be used in moderation where necessary (for example for cooking eggs). While recent media attention has questioned whether saturated fat in meat and dairy (specifically butter) is bad for the heart, a recent study, published in the *British Medical Journal*, found that the danger of saturated fats is real, and concluded that people who eat less of them do in fact have less heart disease. Frank Hu, a co-author of the study, said it 'dispels the notion that "butter is back"'. The bottom line of this study is that 'it is important to focus on replacing saturated fats (which butter is high in), with healthier unsaturated fats or unrefined carbohydrates', which is exactly in line with The Food Effect guidance.

Nut oils

Of the most popular nut oils, walnut oil is rich in heart-healthy omega-3 fatty acids, and hazelnut oil is rich in vitamin E. Unfortunately, heat alters their taste, and they can taste 'burnt' very quickly. They are best drizzled on salads or added to vegetables.

Nuts

Nuts have long been feared as the enemy of weight loss due to their high calorie count – but thankfully, the truth has now largely won out and people are finally coming to their senses about these glorious little wonders, realising that eating nuts does not make you fat. In fact, it's quite the opposite; not only have studies shown that those who consume nuts are slimmer, but their endless health benefits (ranging from improved heart health to glowing skin) are now also undisputed. Here's the low-down on these little nutritional powerhouses.

Good for health

Countless scientific studies have shown that eating nuts can really boost health and prevent illness – most notably, improving general heart health and specifically lowering the risk of heart disease. And the benefits don't end there. A review of twenty-five scientific studies (what's known as a meta-analysis study) led scientists to conclude that eating 70g of nuts per day resulted in lower total cholesterol and lower 'bad' LDL cholesterol. Ironically, it's their high polyunsaturated and monounsaturated fats that lower cholesterol levels in the blood.

Other studies suggest that eating just a handful of nuts each day may help to reduce not only heart disease and high cholesterol, but also high blood pressure, high blood-sugar levels and excess abdominal fat (that is, the metabolic syndrome).

Good for staying slim

Many people think that because nuts are high in calories, they'll inevitably pile on the pounds. However, research shows quite the opposite to be the case. One Spanish study of almost 9,000 adults showed that those who ate nuts at least twice a week had a much lower risk of gaining weight over the next few years compared with those who rarely or never ate them. Another study found that despite having the same calorie intake, adults who included 84g of almonds in their daily diet in place of some of the carbs, had around a 60 per cent greater reduction in weight and body fat after six months compared to those who did not eat them. Bottom line: not only does eating nuts *not* cause weight gain, but it may actually help you lose weight (and stay slim).

Good for training and fitness

Nuts contain the perfect combination of protein, to protect muscle tissue and repair damaged cells, and healthy essential fatty acids, which have incredible anti-inflammatory properties. Consuming some protein before and after a workout has been shown to have beneficial effects. A small amount of pre-exercise protein increases amino acid levels during exercise, which serves as a 'biochemical signal' that tells muscles not to break down protein for fuel. After exercise, consuming protein reduces the negative effects of muscle damage on your ability to exercise the next day. As mentioned previously, the essential fats found in all nuts will further protect your muscles against free-radical damage both during and after training, by strengthening muscle-cell membranes.

The practical bit

Nuts are portable, versatile, nutritious and delicious. If you're looking for the easiest healthy snack to stash in your handbag, briefcase, pocket or office drawer – nuts fit the bill. They are the perfect thing to grab for an instant energy boost during that dreaded mid-afternoon slump. Because of their ideal combination of protein, healthy fats, fibre and low-GI carbs, they promote satiety and prevent you reaching for unhealthy sugar- and fat-laden junk food. Keeping your hunger in check between meals not only keeps your energy levels stable throughout the day, it's also an indispensable weight-loss strategy.

Each nut has its own specific nutrient profile and health benefits, but any nut will offer heart-healthy fats, vitamin E (a

critical antioxidant), fibre, protein and a host of other beneficial nutrients. Any nut is a great choice, as long as you stick to
the portions listed below, as well as those laid out in The Food
Effect meal plans.

While all the evidence is in favour of nuts for healthy weight
control, you definitely can't go eating a whole big bag each day (I
discuss this in more detail on page 95). Keep portions to around
30g per day (or as specified in The Food Effect snack options),
and ideally stick to unsalted varieties. If you're out and about
or buying for work or travelling, buy nuts in pre-portioned bags
(30–50g), or do your own portioning at home, into small Ziploc
bags or Tupperware containers, once you've stocked up on a big
bag.

The numbers of nuts that make up a 30g portion are roughly:
24 almonds, 18 cashew nuts, 28 peanuts, 14 walnuts and 49 pistachio nuts. Note that portion sizes might be smaller if specified
with fruit in your Food Effect options and meal plans.

Avocados

As well as being extremely delicious, these are a wonderful source
of the healthy monounsaturated fats, which have been shown
to help lower blood pressure, and are extremely good for your
heart. They have been shown to improve 'bad' LDL cholesterol
and reduce the risk of heart disease in people who are overweight
and obese. They are also a rich source of fibre, which helps to
control blood-sugar levels, as well as potassium, which helps
lower blood pressure.

While it's commonly known that bananas are a good source
of potassium, avocados actually contain even more of this essential nutrient. Half an avocado contains more potassium than a
medium-sized banana – so you won't even be missing out, as
bananas are a no-no on The Food Effect diet (see page 43).

Avocados have also been shown to help people feel fuller for
longer and stave off the munchies between lunch and dinner. A

recent study in *Nutrition Journal* found that overweight adults who ate half an avocado at lunch had a 40 per cent decrease in the desire to eat again over the next three hours – and for some, the feeling of fullness lasted a whole five hours. Because avocados are so creamy, they help to satisfy cravings.

Guacamole (made from avocados) is a great option when you're craving a high-fat treat. Avocados also help to strengthen your immune system, being rich in glutathione – a powerful antioxidant, detoxifier and free-radical scavenger. Lastly but certainly not least importantly, avocados help to keep your skin, nails and hair healthy.

Losing weight while looking and feeling your best

The Food Effect approach to fats and diet in general is not just aimed at weight loss; it is also targeted at improving overall health, including heart health and disease prevention. It can be backed up by the latest research, which shows that consuming plenty of vegetables, nuts and olive oil is more effective than using drugs such as statins in treating heart disease. Patients who stuck to a Mediterranean diet were a third less likely to die early than those who ate more red meat and butter, Italian researchers found. A diet rich in fish and fruit has long been known to be good for the heart, and the latest results confirm this. Those who ate mainly along Mediterranean lines (higher in monounsaturated fats, and low in saturated fats such as those from meat and butter) were 37 per cent less likely to die during the study than those who ate a diet heavier in saturated fats, and that was after adjusting for age, sex, class and exercise.

Simple signs that suggest you may be lacking in essential fats are dry skin, constipation, poor wound healing, frequent infections, inflammation of the joints and small bumps on the backs of your upper arms. You may be saying goodbye to many of these problems once you start eating The Food Effect way.

As you can see, The Food Effect diet encourages you to eat from a wide variety of healthy fat sources, while reducing saturated and trans-fats, for both health optimisation and weight-loss reasons. All the good fats are included in the correct amounts in the meal plans. You certainly won't be going 'fat-free' with The Food Effect diet, but you'll be relying on the healthiest choices of fats, thereby promoting weight loss and keeping you full and satiated.

CHAPTER 7

Snacking and Overeating

Banish cravings, avoid overeating and master your self-control

By now you'll have read the fundamentals of The Food Effect way of life and The Food Effect rules. These will help ensure you eat healthily, minimise hunger and cravings, and keep your blood-sugar levels stable, to achieve your target weight and maintain your health and weight over the long term. However, even with a practical, easy to follow meal plan and manageable set of rules, there will still be times when you feel you just 'need' that bar of chocolate, or want to eat way more than you should.

While I do see the occasional client who never gets cravings or the urge to overeat, this is certainly not the norm. Although I can assure you that The Food Effect diet will leave you feeling more satisfied and less deprived than other diets out there, I know that having a few additional tactics – both practical and psychological – will go a long way in helping you to banish cravings, avoid overeating and master your self-control.

Why do we overeat?

We've all overeaten at some point (if you never have, you're an admirable, rare human being). It can happen for a range of reasons: boredom (shown to be one of the most common reasons), loneliness, sadness, stress, anxiety and access to large volumes of tempting food, to name just a few. If you overeat only very occasionally, for example at a festive meal or special party, then you are able to take control and get back on track with your healthy eating plan the next day, that's quite normal and won't be a major issue in your weight-loss journey.

Unfortunately, far too many of us overeat on a regular (if not daily) basis, and are gaining weight, or not losing it, as a result. If you regularly go to bed bursting with food, or finish a meal feeling uncomfortably full, now might be the time to take a closer look at why you are overeating and develop ways to control it.

Overeating on a regular basis is often strongly linked to our mood. Stress, sadness, frustration or any unresolved emotion can cause you to turn to food for comfort. This behavioural response may have been taught to us by parents or carers who offer food, usually of the sweet sugary type, to soothe a crying injured infant or a sad teen, for example. Or it may be self-taught – we remember the pleasure that we instantaneously experience when we eat certain foods (think your favourite tub of ice-cream), then seek out this sensation again to ease emotional pain. Unfortunately, while food does temporarily numb emotional pain or fill an emotional void, the pain or void is not fixed, so the habit of overeating may continue for days, weeks and months, if not years, while we continue to reinforce this short-term reward system that we have developed. Additionally, it is not difficult to overeat. The fullness mechanism in the body is nowhere near as tightly regulated as hunger is. It's far easier to override your 'fullness' signal, especially when high-calorie, high-fat and high-sugar food is readily available, than it is to ignore your hunger signals for a significant amount of time.

Being aware of when overeating is most likely to occur for you, in your day-to-day life, is a crucial part of taking control of overeating, as is learning to listen to your body when it comes to the volume of food it needs. If you have been overeating for a long period of time, this may be especially difficult, if not impossible for you to do naturally on your own. That's why The Food Effect attack phase and lifestyle meal plans and options have been designed and laid out with all portions specified for you – all you have to do is follow them, and I can guarantee you won't be overeating.

How to take control

1. Know your high-risk situations These are different for each person. You may overeat socially, or perhaps only in private; you may do it during that mid-afternoon slump; or you may not be able to control late-night cravings even after you've had dinner. Whatever the case may be, the chances are that there is a specific time or situation when you are most likely to overeat. Once you identify what times are 'risky' for you, it's simple to develop strategies to manage these situations (see more on this in the tips to control cravings and avoid overeating, page 88). Focus on implementing these strategies at the times you are most vulnerable. You may find you need to have your mid-afternoon snack close to the time you are heading out to dinner so you don't overeat when you're out at a restaurant, or have a cut-off time for stopping to eat in the evening if late-night snacking is your problem. Whatever your 'high-risk' overeating time is, the key is to implement some management strategies for it then.

2. Get in tune with your hunger and fullness signals Many of us eat so much or so often (or both), that we can't even remember the last time we felt really truly hungry. I'm not suggesting you should let yourself reach the point of feeling starving (in fact it is a Food Effect rule that you do *not* do this), but if you can't recognise true hunger, it's also difficult to gauge when you are actually full. For many of us, it may only be at the point where we feel 'stuffed' or uncomfortable. If this is the case, try paying closer attention to the point at which you start to feel full and satisfied. Usually, it's a mouthful or two before the actual 'full' feeling, especially as it takes the stomach at least 10–20 minutes to register true fullness, and even longer for the food you eat to reach the end of your intestine where more satiety hormones are released. So give it some time before deciding that you need seconds. Chew each mouthful slowly, and place your cutlery down between mouthfuls. This will help you to gauge how your body is feeling, so you won't eat like a machine on autopilot – and as I said earlier (see page 29), eating slowly will also ensure that your brain actually registers when you've eaten enough food, before it's too late.

3. Tailor your environment Quite simply, if it's not there, you won't eat it. If you keep a steady supply of tempting treats at home or at work, then it's quite natural that when you're feeling bored, tired, stressed or down, you'll eat them. Keep away from the pile of sweets, chocolates, biscuits or birthday cake that colleagues bring to work. If you tell yourself those things are off-limits for you (they are all in the 'stay away' column, see page 24, after all, and for good reason), you won't be caught in the overindulgence trap. Once you start with those foods, they just trigger cravings for more unhealthy, sugary or fatty foods, so it's easier not to start eating them in the first place.

4. Learn to compensate While, ideally, none of us would ever overeat or overindulge from now on, that's highly unlikely and also unnecessary – after all, what's a birthday without some cake? So, one strategy for when you *do* overindulge is

to *compensate*. By this I definitely don't mean starving yourself the next day or even skipping a meal, but as I discuss on
page 99, you might want to choose a salad or soup (or any of
the options from the attack phase plan) for a meal, rather than
a steak and sweet potato – even though that's allowed in the
lifestyle phase once you're on that, after the first four weeks).
Learning to compensate healthily will help you feel physically
better when you have overeaten, and help balance your overall
intake so that the occasional indulgence doesn't hamper your
weight-loss goals.

Top tips to control cravings and avoid overeating

Here are a few simple strategies to banish those cravings and
avoid unnecessary overeating or snacking.

- **Avoid your triggers** You crave what you eat ... so change
  what you're eating to the *right* foods (see 'eat this' options
  in Chapter 2) to weaken your cravings for the bad stuff. As
  I've said, the foods in the 'stay away' columns in Chapter 2
  are labelled 'stay away' for good reasons – they do nothing to
  benefit your health or weight, or to help banish cravings.
- **If you don't want to eat it, don't keep it in the house.**
- **Put leftovers away immediately.**
- **Avoid buffet and 'all-you-can-eat' restaurants** – especially if
  you find this type of scenario tempting; this is just a sure-fire
  ticket to overeating unnecessarily.
- **Allow yourself to indulge within limits** Practise portion
  control or a healthier indulgence in moderation (like a few
  squares of good-quality dark chocolate, or a decadent dessert
  made with healthy ingredients ... yes such things do exist).
  See snacks and sweet treat recipes (page 234) for ideas.
- **Plan ahead** If you know there's an upcoming situation where
  you are going to indulge, allocate calories and factor them

into your eating plan that day (but don't go there hungry – you'll just set yourself up for disaster). My best advice would be: when you do go for a treat and allow yourself the odd indulgence, make it pleasurable by choosing something you truly enjoy, and savour every bite.

- **Schedule snacking** If you find yourself constantly tempted to have that chocolate bar and eventually feel so hungry you can't resist it, make sure you never skip lunch or your mid-afternoon snack, and try to schedule it before the time you get ravenous. So if, say, by 4.30 p.m. you feel ravenous every day, tell yourself that on any given day 3.30 p.m. is your snack time. Buy a healthy snack ahead of time or have something with you (at work or in your bag), so you don't get the urge to go out and buy that giant chocolate bar.

- **Focus on protein and fibre for a filling snack** There's nothing wrong with having a snack in between meals – in fact it's encouraged and specified in The Food Effect rules and meal plans, even during the attack phase. Our bodies typically need something to eat about every 3–4 hours. For the most satiating and energy-boosting snacks, choose options that contain both protein and fibre, for example an apple with a tablespoon of peanut butter or a handful of almonds, or hummus with carrot sticks. There is a long list of options on page 175, so you don't need to think too much about this one; it's all there for you. Adding more fibre and protein to your snacks slows digestion and ensures better blood sugar regulation, making you less likely to reach for unhealthy snacks and junk food.

- **Go nuts (in moderation)** If despite having eaten enough, you still have a strong urge to snack, drink two glasses of water and eat a 30g serving of nuts (around 12 walnuts, 16 cashew nuts, 20 almonds, 28 peanuts or 49 pistachios), then reassess how you feel. Nuts are my all-time favourite snack, which I recommend to clients, as they fulfil the criteria of the tip above in one neat package. Nuts are packed with an amazing profile of healthy fats, fibre, protein and micronutrients (vitamins and minerals), while satisfying hunger cravings. If you're out and about and suddenly feel ravenous between meals, bags of nuts are a staple in many food shops and make an extremely healthy choice – far better than crisps or chocolate. A single serving of nuts contains only about 130 calories, but beware of those jumbo-sized bags that can contain a whopping ten servings! One solution is to pack your own nuts as single servings in a small snack bag or Tupperware container. One serving of nuts is about 30g, but remember that the number of pieces varies by nut, as specified above. Pistachios are a great choice because cracking each one open takes time, allowing you to enjoy them for longer.

- **Sip something steamy** If you're craving a chocolate bar or your stomach is rumbling mid-morning or afternoon and there's no healthy food in sight, try a hot skinny latte instead. Caffeine in moderation has health benefits (or you can go for decaffeinated), and you'll be getting protein and calcium from the milk, while avoiding all the calories, sugar and unhealthy fats found in junk chocolate. Herbal teas are another great option for any time of day – there are many delicious sweet flavours on the market that are perfect for a mid-morning or mid-afternoon pick-me-up, as well as in the late evening when the munchies strike.

- **Stay well hydrated** You've heard this one before but it deserves reiteration. *Drink, drink, drink.* And by this I mean water. Often when we think we're hungry, we're actually just thirsty, so make sure you drink plenty of water throughout the day, as well as 1–2 glasses *before* every meal or snack you have. Symptoms of dehydration can mimic the feelings of hunger, so before you reach for a 250-calorie chocolate bar, drink a bottle of zero-calorie water. Water aids weight loss by helping your kidneys flush out excess toxins and chemicals, which may be slowing down your metabolism. If you have difficulty drinking enough plain water – which should be around 2 litres a day – herbal teas, green tea and lemon in hot water are all just as good.

- **If you're eating due to tiredness, take a power nap instead.**
- **Brush your teeth and gargle with mouthwash** if you're going to eat unnecessarily, especially late at night. You'll be less likely to go and eat more food with a clean mouth and the taste of mint on your tongue.
- **Distract yourself and let stress go with other techniques** We all tend to snack when we are bored, so find other ways to stay busy. Keep occupied around the house, or even take up a new hobby. Taking your mind off food will help to reduce unnecessary mindless snacking. Read a book or file some papers to keep your hands and mind busy; or take a walk after dinner. Cravings usually last around ten minutes, so find a non-food-related activity to pass the time and take your mind off food. Bored? Call a friend, read a magazine or a good book, or do some tidying or organising. Angry? Try to do some exercise to get rid of the anger in a way that empowers rather than disempowers you. The burst of activity will also release endorphins (feel-good hormones) that make you feel happy and less stressed. If you can hold off from craving-induced eating for ten minutes, you may well overcome the urge altogether.
- **Dodge the comfort-food trap** This is especially pertinent when winter comes around. It's tempting to curl up on the sofa and binge on stodgy carbs and sweet treats, but far from making you feel good, typical so-called 'comfort food' can leave you tired, lethargic and moody. Instead, get your sweet fix from fruit or any of The Food Effect Energy Balls (see recipes, pages 241–42), which raise your serotonin levels naturally.
- **Get your soup on** When you crave comfort food, heat up a large bowl of soup made with lots of vegetables and beans. It's flavourful, hearty, high in satiating protein, fibre and nutrition, and low in fat and calories – the perfect thing to keep you feeling full and satisfied (starting on page 224),

Snacking staples

Stock up on the healthy snacking staples listed below (and refer to the list of snack options in The Food Effect meal plans and options). Make sure you have these foods on hand at home or at work, to avoid the urge to seek out a sugary chocolate bar or bag of crisps instead.

Raw vegetables

Crunchy vegetables can help ease stress and cravings in a purely mechanical way. Munching celery or carrot sticks can ward off tension by helping to release a clenched jaw. Whenever you feel the urge to snack, but know you've eaten enough and just want something to munch on, chew on some celery sticks. Keep a jar or container full of them submerged in cold water, for a refreshing crunchy snack.

When you're looking for something a bit more substantial, pair your chosen raw veg with a serving of hummus.

Fresh fruit

Fresh fruit never fails. You can't go wrong snacking on fruit such as disease-fighting blueberries, apples and oranges, which have been shown to reduce the risk of heart disease and certain cancers. Additionally, the potassium, magnesium and calcium in most fresh produce have been proven to help lower blood pressure. Ready-cut fresh fruit and fruit salads are sold in most food shops and supermarkets – perfect for when you're on the go and in need of a sweet fix. Berries are a particularly good option, as they are very low in calories and sugar, yet their sweetness helps to replace sugar cravings and leaves you feeling fresh and satisfied.

Dark chocolate

This type of chocolate contains two compounds that can lower stress levels – anandamide, which binds to receptors in the brain that produce feelings of euphoria, and phenylethylamine (PEA), a substance naturally found in our nervous systems that is released throughout the brain when we fall in love. If you fancy a sweet treat, dark chocolate (anything that is at least 70 per cent cocoa) is sure to satisfy your cravings and has also been shown to protect against cardiovascular disease and help lower blood pressure. It is far better than having sweet snacks that contain large amounts of refined sugars, which deplete B vitamins that are needed for energy, and leave you feeling unsatisfied and in need of more sweet sugary foods. The flavonols found in cocoa – the main constituent of dark chocolate – also improve circulation and increase blood flow to the brain, which helps you think and see more clearly. Opt for non-dairy dark chocolate, because it contains the highest amount of powerful antioxidants. Limit the portion size to 2–4 squares a day for a snack. See meal plans for portions and specified options incorporating dark chocolate.

Oatcakes

Because oats are so high in fibre, few things take longer for your stomach to digest, allowing a sustained release of the feel-good neurotransmitter serotonin. Oats, in the form of porridge, are therefore included as part of your breakfast options, but oat-*cakes* make a great snacking choice, too (as specified in The Food Effect snack options). Studies have shown that including five servings of whole grains a day as part of a calorie-controlled diet can help you lose abdominal fat and lower your levels of C-reactive protein (CRP), a predictor of heart disease, stroke and diabetes.

Low-fat dairy foods

Including dairy foods such as skimmed milk or low-fat natural yoghurts, as part of a balanced diet, has been shown to aid weight loss (see Chapter 4). Additionally, 1,000mg of calcium a day will help you to maintain bone mass when trying to lose weight. Calcium can also reduce muscle spasms and soothe tension, and in fact skimmed and semi-skimmed milk are higher in calcium and protein than full fat. It has also been shown to reduce stressful PMS symptoms such as mood swings, anxiety and irritability, which all do nothing to help with emotional eating. So a skinny latte or a low-fat natural yoghurt, for example, are great snacks.

Cottage cheese

Low-fat cottage cheese is extremely filling and weighs in at less than 200 calories for a whole tub (about a cupful). In addition to being high in protein and low in carbohydrates, cottage cheese also contains probiotics, the healthy bacteria that help improve your digestion. It's also packed with calcium, and as mentioned, calcium-rich diets have been found to aid weight loss.

Oranges

The magic nutrient here is vitamin C. A German study in the journal *Psychopharmacology* found that vitamin C helps reduce stress and return blood pressure and cortisol back to normal levels following a stressful situation (raised cortisol is linked with weight gain and fat storage). Vitamin C is also well known for strengthening the immune system. So next time you're feeling stressed-out about something, go peel yourself an orange.

Nuts

It is a shame that some people avoid them as they are high in calories, because if eaten in the right amounts, they are definitely one of the best snacks out there. They provide essential healthy fats and omega-3s, which are crucial for the brain, improve circulation and prevent inflammation. These will keep hunger at bay for several hours until your next meal. Snacking on nuts may help you shed pounds and reduce abdominal fat. Researchers have found that people who ate almonds as part of a low-calorie diet for six months lost 18 per cent of their body weight compared with those who did not. Additionally, monounsaturated fats found in nuts have been shown to lower harmful LDL cholesterol levels, while increasing the good HDL cholesterol that benefits your body. All nuts are a great snack that can be portioned ahead of time for when you get hungry. Because nuts are calorific, make sure you measure your serving (see portion sizes on page 81). While all nuts make a great snack, a few deserve a special mention:

Almonds

Almonds are packed full of B vitamins, which make you more resilient during bouts of stress, and vitamin E, which helps bolster your immune system. To get the benefits, snack on about twenty almonds every day. Another way to get your fix is to eat some almond butter, although make sure you go for the sugar-free variety and stick to a small serving.

Pistachios and walnuts

Both these will help keep your heart from racing when things get stressful. Research has shown that eating a handful of pistachios a day lowers blood pressure so that your heart doesn't have to work overtime. Walnuts have the most antioxidant power of all varieties of nut and are packed with magnesium and healthy omega-3 fatty acids. Walnuts have also been found to lower blood pressure, both at rest and under stress. As well as making a great snack, chopped walnuts can be sprinkled over salads, cereal or porridge.

Hummus

This makes a healthy energy-boosting snack that is sure to satisfy any creamy-salty cravings. It's a great energy booster when paired with vegetables like red peppers, carrots and cucumbers.

Avocados

One of the best ways to reduce high blood pressure is to consume enough potassium, and avocados actually have more of this essential nutrient than bananas. Yes, half an avocado has more potassium than a medium-sized banana. The monounsaturated fats found in avocados also help to lower blood pressure and are extremely heart healthy. Guacamole can be a great option when stress makes you crave a high-fat treat.

A word on visualisation

Visualising your future self can play a huge role in developing self-control with food. We've all been there before – opening the jar of peanut butter to have 'just one teaspoon', or that tub of Häagen-Dazs sitting in our freezer for 'just one scoop'; but, before you know it, you're scraping the last remnant from the jar or have reached the bottom of the ice-cream tub.

The 'just one' mentality is about as difficult to master as the Rubik's Cube. When it comes to eating well (that is, sticking to the right foods *and* the right quantities), most people will admit that self-control is the hardest part. But here's the good news – science has cracked the code to impulse-proofing eating habits. New research from the University of Zurich postulates that being able to focus on your future needs is one way to achieve self-control. The researchers found that if you bypass your 'present self' to love your 'future self' you can resist that in-the-moment temptation (so it is possible to stop yourself from finishing that tub of ice-cream!).

So how do you fend off your self-indulgent urges and stay in touch with your future desires? Here are my tips for doing this:

- Place reminders of your health goals in plain sight to help you visualise the person you want to be. For example, you may want to write on a big Post-It note: 'I never feel good after over-indulging in junk food and I don't want to be a person who always craves sugar,' or 'Sugar makes me feel tired, lethargic and moody; I don't want it to be a staple part of my diet.'
- Keep your long-term achievement of health at the forefront of your mind by writing motivational notes and creating an inspiration board. You can do this by hand, having a board on Pinterest, or saving inspirational pictures and quotes on your phone and browsing through them regularly.

By doing the above, you'll create your own strong vision of your ideal healthy self (remember, we are all different and it's important to be realistic and not make unhealthy comparisons with others), so when that salted caramel ice-cream seems a little too appealing, you can check back in with the needs of your 'future self' that you have pictured so strongly in your mind, and find the strength to say 'No thanks, maybe some other time!'

CHAPTER 8

Dining Out Done Right

How to make eating out healthy and enjoyable

Eating out has become so common in our culture these days. Restaurants were once visited on special occasions but now, according to the National Restaurant Association, almost half of all adults eat at a restaurant or order a takeaway every day, for convenience, variety or taste. People are looking for fast, easy and tasty food to fit their busy lifestyles. Whether it's in sit-down restaurants, food courts, takeaways, office cafeterias or hospital canteens, dining out has become an integral part of everyday life, and there are abundant choices everywhere you turn. Thankfully, by following The Food Effect rules and tips when dining out, you can still lose weight and maintain a healthy social life.

While ready-made healthy options are becoming a lot more common, and there are usually several healthy options to choose from when dining out, there are still many more 'bad' choices available, and a lot of opportunities to go wrong and ruin your waistline. This doesn't mean you shouldn't eat out and need to become a social recluse just because you're leading a healthy lifestyle and watching your weight. The Food Effect approach is all about enjoying life and living normally. The Food Effect diet is based on the approach I took in devising plans to suit busy Londoners, who don't have much time to spend preparing home-cooked meals in the kitchen. Eating out can be healthy *and* enjoyable – this chapter guides you on everything you need to know about dining out (or ordering in), done right. If you *do* prefer to cook and prepare your own meals, the recipes in Chapter 13 will give you everything you need.

Before getting on to specific types of food and restaurants, as well as tips for eating when travelling or at an airport, here are my general tips for eating healthfully when dining out.

Before you order

- If you're nervous about maintaining your healthy eating plan, think ahead, do some research, and plan where you're going to eat or order from. Check out the restaurant's website and consider what meal options are available. Look for restaurants or takeaway options with a wide range of menu items. With so many places available, you don't need to go for that one Chinese option with only greasy, fried food.
- Plan ahead. If you know you're going to be eating a large meal in the evening, consider your food choices for that entire day, not just that night – perhaps have a slightly lighter breakfast and lunch. I definitely don't suggest that you skip meals or arrive at dinner hungry (that goes against The Food Effect rules), but you might choose a healthy salad that day instead of a heavier sandwich, for lunch.
- If you are familiar with the menu, decide what to order before entering the restaurant. This tactic will help you to avoid any tempting foods that may not be particularly healthy.
- If you are trying a new restaurant, take time to look over the menu and make careful selections in order to avoid making

unhealthy decisions. Some restaurant menus may have a special section for 'healthier' choices, or options such as 'light' cheese, whole-wheat pasta or brown rice for sushi.

- Pay attention to restaurant menu terms for clues as to fat and calorie content. Baked, braised, broiled, grilled, poached, roasted and steamed all imply less fat and calories than battered, buttered, fried, creamed, crispy, sautéed and so on. Avoid or limit the latter choices as much as possible.

When you order

- As mentioned above, stick to ordering baked, braised, broiled, grilled, poached, roasted or steamed foods.
- In place of fries or chips, choose a side salad, steamed vegetables or a baked potato
- Order vegetable side dishes (or potatoes) baked, steamed, boiled or roasted rather than fried. Ask the waiter to omit any butter, cream or creamy sauces, or ask them to put them on the side.
- If you are ordering a soup, stick to broth-based soups such as minestrone or chicken noodle soup, or non-creamy vegetable soups such as gazpacho.
- Refer to the tables in Chapter 2, and stick to foods in the 'eat this' (or 'be careful') columns, avoiding anything that comes under 'stay away'. So, for example, choose chicken or fish rather than fatty meats; remove skin from chicken and all visible fat from any red meat (which you can order occasionally once you're on the lifestyle phase).
- When choosing or assembling a salad, avoid items like grated hard cheeses, creamy dressings (unless specified as low fat or light) and fried croutons.
- For salads, always order the dressing on the side so that you can control how much you use – and use it sparingly. Better yet, use a squeeze of lemon instead of a dressing, or try balsamic, apple cider or rice vinegar.

- Ask the waiter about ingredients or preparation methods for any dishes you're unsure about. It's OK to make special requests, but keep them simple (remember, The Food Effect is all about encouraging normality). For example, it's perfectly reasonable and sensible to ask for a baked potato or extra side salad in place of French fries; no mayonnaise or bacon on your sandwich; and sauces and dressings on the side.
- If you're getting a sandwich made up for you, boost the bulk and nutrition by adding tomato, lettuce, peppers or other vegetables. Choose lean protein fillings such as tuna, smoked salmon, egg, turkey or chicken on whole-grain bread. Ask for mustard, ketchup or salsa (all allowed on The Food Effect diet), and avoid butter, margarine and full-fat mayonnaise.

During the meal

- Avoid eating too much before your meal even arrives. So no bread and olive oil, crisps or cashew nuts – wait for your meal to be served instead. Once you get stuck into the bread basket, it's not hard to eat two or three pieces before dinner, and that can be equal to a whole meal's worth of calories before you even get to your main course.
- Avoid 'all-you-can-eat' specials, buffets and unlimited salad bars if you tend to eat too much at this type of meal. If you do choose a buffet, fill up on salads and vegetables first. Take no more than two trips and use a small plate.
- Eat lower calorie food first. If everyone is ordering a starter, a vegetable-based soup (rather than a creamy one) or fresh salad is a good choice. Avoid anything deep fried or battered. Follow it with a light main course.
- Limit the amount of alcohol you drink to no more than one drink per evening out (more specifics on alcohol in Chapter 9).
- Tempted by sweet, creamy desserts? During your first four weeks on the attack phase these are a complete no-no. You

may, however, order fresh fruit without whipped cream, ice-cream or a topping. Another great trick is to drink more. By that I mean order a cup of (decaf) coffee or herbal tea at the end of the meal, so that you're occupied while the other diners are tucking into that tiramisu or hot chocolate cake. You'll be less tempted to eat dessert if you're busy sipping your tea and making good conversation. Once you're at the lifestyle phase, I'd still advise you to avoid calorific desserts (they don't provide much in the way of nutrition). If you must (and if the other diners agree!), order one dessert with enough forks for everyone at the table to have a bite. Alternatively, sorbet is not a bad choice – while it does contain sugar, it doesn't include fat and it's not too high in calories.

• Take home leftovers. If you can't finish your extra-large sandwich or pasta dish, you don't need to eat it just to avoid wasting it; take half home for another meal or lunch the next day. Any restaurant will be more than happy to pack up your leftovers if you ask – that way you get two meals for the price of one *and* don't ruin your waistline.

Specific types of cuisine

Italian

As discussed earlier, owing to low-carb diet crazes and bad science, foods like pasta and pizza have gained a bad reputation, and those looking to lose weight would usually never dream of touching these foods (or if they did, would guiltily assume they had 'broken their diet'). Yet in Italy, people eat pasta daily without the country having the same obesity rates as those in the UK and the US, and on The Food Effect diet, you can enjoy them too. Here's how . . .

Staying slim while enjoying pasta

My aim here is to bust a few myths. Pasta is *not* the weight-loss enemy it's often made out to be. There is every reason why you can eat this versatile carb without piling on the pounds (while gaining valuable nutritional benefits in the process). Here is the how and why.

When I suggest incorporating pasta into my clients' diets I am often met with an incredulous stare and the response: 'But isn't pasta fattening?' The truth is, I hate this question. No – pasta itself is not '*fattening*'. Pasta is a 'low-fat' food with just 1.5g of fat per 75g serving. It's usually the specific type, how much you eat and what goes on your pasta that makes it a potential diet disaster (think big bowls of white pasta laden with thick cream sauce and yellow cheese). So I'm certainly not giving you free rein to eat all types of pasta in vast quantities.

Rule 1 White pasta is out – whole-grain pasta is in (where possible). Whole grains (like oats, barley and brown rice) contain fibre, protein, healthy fats and an abundance of vitamins and minerals. Good-quality whole-wheat and brown rice pasta provide a good dose of these nutrients. The fibre and protein in whole-wheat pasta means that a smaller portion will keep you fuller for longer, and ensure your blood-sugar levels remain stable. Whether you go for whole-wheat or brown rice pasta (which is gluten-free), both have several further benefits.

1. A cup of cooked whole-wheat pasta provides around a quarter of your daily fibre requirements. As mentioned above, increased fibre helps you feel fuller (on fewer calories), thereby aiding and boosting weight loss.
2. Both whole-wheat and brown rice pasta are good sources of B vitamins such as thiamin (essential for energy production, carbohydrate metabolism and nerve-cell function), riboflavin

(needed for healthy skin turnover and maintenance), and niacin (needed in fat, cholesterol and carbohydrate metabolism, and the production of many body compounds, including sex and adrenal hormones).

3. Pasta is one of the most versatile foods around – with countless available types (like spaghetti, penne, fettuccine, tagliatelle, macaroni, ravioli and lasagne) and numerous ways to serve up pasta dishes (think added vegetables), you will never be stuck for options. It's also the perfect match for tomato sauces, which are rich in the super-antioxidant lycopene.

If there's no whole-wheat pasta on the menu, there's no need to avoid ordering pasta (unless you're on the attack phase, where pasta is out for four weeks), but make sure you stick to the next rule.

Rule 2 Be careful how *much* pasta you eat. While pasta itself is low fat and nutritious, it does contain a reasonable amount of calories. This is not necessarily a bad thing, but it does need to be taken into account in determining how much to eat. A 75g serving (uncooked) provides around 270 calories – this is perfectly suitable for a main meal (with additions), but it's often hard to stop at just one serving, and the bowls you get in a restaurant usually contain at least two servings. Spaghetti as a main dish can weigh in at a whopping 1,000 calories, more than half your daily calorie allowance. A simple way to tackle this sensibly is to eat half and get the waiter to pack up the other half, or share a main-course portion with a friend or partner. Another good trick I often share with my clients is to fill half your bowl with vegetables – either fresh spinach or salad leaves, or steamed green beans or broccoli. This works because volume plays a large role in determining how satisfied we are from a meal. If we've had a large, full bowl of 'real' food, we'll feel just as satisfied even though half of it was low-calorie vegetables and the other half pasta.

Rule 3 Watch what goes *on* your pasta. Thick, creamy, buttery and cheesy sauces are out – they are guaranteed to add hundreds of calories and grams of fat to a meal. Opt for tomato-based sauces wherever possible, and if you must have cheese, stick to just a light sprinkle of Parmesan.

Staying slim while enjoying pizza

You probably never thought you'd hear a doctor or nutritionist tell you that pizza can actually make a healthy balanced meal, but I'm going to do just that. If you consider its components, pizza has the potential to pack in plenty of goodness. Healthy carbohydrates from the base (especially if it is whole wheat), high levels of the cancer-fighting antioxidant lycopene in the tomato sauce, plus protein, calcium and fats from a light serving of cheese, and endless other sources of nutrients if you load up your pizza with vegetable toppings such as red onion, peppers, mushrooms and corn, mean that the bad reputation given to pizza can be a thing of the past.

Of course, let's be honest here – a thick-crust, cheese-laden pizza is far from a health food. Although this does vary, one slice of a large, thick-crust pizza contains 300–400 calories, and an average 16g of fat – 7g of which is saturated – as a result of the oil-glistening cheese. But if you order right, there's no need to deprive yourself any longer. So here are some suggestions for ways in which you can enjoy a pizza while keeping the experience waistline-friendly.

1. **Half please** Unless you're an active teenage boy or man, you generally only need half a pizza for a decent-sized meal (with a side salad or preceded by a vegetable soup). To prevent overeating and the excess calories that come along with it, either share a pizza with a fellow diner, or take the other half home for later (because, let's be honest, who would ever turn down leftover pizza?). It can be reheated, or even enjoyed cold the next day.

2. **Stick to smart sides** They might be tasty, but side orders like French fries, onion rings and garlic bread are loaded with calories and unhealthy fats. So keep your sides light yet filling, by sticking to things like a side salad or vegetables.

3. **Skip the cheese** Eating cheese-less vegetable pizza is an easy way to cut out a great deal of calories and unhealthy saturated fat. A good 'saucy' pizza topped with veggies is absolutely delicious and far from bland and boring. If it *really* doesn't seem like 'real pizza' to you and it won't 'hit the spot', ask for a light sprinkling of cheese rather than the usual heavy-handed serving. It will still amount to fewer calories than a typical pizza packed with cheese, and will allow those delicious vegetables to take centre stage instead.

4. **Thin is in** Thin-crust pizza is far lower in carbs and calories than those deep-dish pizza pies. It's also far more authentic and Italian in style, so be sure to order thin crust wherever possible.

5. **Go whole-wheat** If available, order a whole-wheat crust. It's much higher in fibre and protein than white, so you feel fuller from less and your body won't turn it straight into sugars and fat. It'll also help keep your blood-sugar levels stable and you feeling fuller for longer. If it's not an option, a thin-crust pizza made with white flour, loaded with veg but with minimal cheese, is still a healthy and balanced option.

6. **When in doubt, blot it out** You might want to save this one for home or for when you have no other choice and are presented with an oil-glistening, cheese-laden slice, but with slices *that* greasy and no other option, you can probably do with all the help you can get. So while there's no way of knowing exactly how many calories you save, if you can do so discretely, try blotting the oil on top of your pizza with a napkin – you'll probably save yourself a good few grams of artery-clogging saturated fat.

Yes, there'll always be those who are willing to order a salad while everyone else devours their pizza and who would never dream of touching a slice, but that's not the approach I advocate. Eating should be pleasurable and enjoyable – especially on occasions when you're dining out or ordering in.

Now that you know my pasta and pizza rules, you can go ahead and enjoy these foods guilt-free, The Food Effect way – rest assured, they will not cause you to pile on the pounds.

Chinese

Chinese food in the West caters to our taste for fried food and heavy, meat-based entrées, rather than the healthy grain and vegetable-based dishes traditionally found in China, where portions of meat are modest.

When choosing what to order in a Chinese restaurant, steer clear of fried dishes such as spring rolls, seaweed, sticky ribs, fried rice and sesame chicken, which pack thousands of calories and a whopping amount of unhealthy fat. Also avoid anything described as 'sweet and sour', as this ultimately means 'coated in a sugary sauce (and sometimes batter too) and fried'. Stick to low-fat dishes that are stir-fried or steamed, and packed with vegetables and lean protein (such as chicken or fish). If steamed vegetables or rice seem bland, order a stir-fried dish and mix it with the steamed side dish (such as broccoli or green beans and mangetout). The sauce from the stir-fry adds flavour to the steamed food, while having a steamed option reduces the overall calorie and fat content provided by two stir-fried dishes together, without any compromise on taste.

Japanese (sushi)

Nowadays, sushi is becoming available almost everywhere you turn – from Japanese restaurants to supermarkets; grocery stores to local bakeries. While it can provide a perfectly balanced and filling meal, sushi can also be a diet disaster if the wrong choices are made. Many people assume that opting for sushi is a guaranteed 'healthy option'. While this may be true sometimes, it's certainly not always the case.

I'm often asked by clients whether they can eat sushi, what they should order, how much and so on. A sushi meal, for example some sashimi and/or a basic cucumber/avocado roll, can weigh in at a measly 200–300 calories or, at the other end of the spectrum, top 1,000 calories – think deep-fried tempura rolls. So while unfortunately there's no simple answer and it's difficult to give a set quantity, what you order, and how much of it, is what makes the difference, as is the context in which it is being eaten (for example as a starter, or as your main meal). Health-wise, you need to know quite a bit when making your sushi choices, so before you order and get stuck in, bear in mind these simple tips for eating sushi and staying slim.

1. Power up with protein and healthy fats When choosing sushi as your main meal, make sure you incorporate a decent amount of protein. While a cucumber roll may seem like the 'diet-friendly' option, and indeed will be lower in calories than fish, you need protein to provide satiety and sustenance to your meal. **Salmon** and **tuna** are among the leanest, highest quality proteins you can eat, and both are rich in heart-healthy omega-3 fatty acids. If you eat sushi daily or on a very regular basis, try not to overdo it on the amount of fish (especially tuna) you consume by including vegetarian rolls to help reduce your intake of mercury. Women who are pregnant or breastfeeding should limit their fish and seafood intake to around 360g per week (a 180g portion twice a week), and avoid raw fish altogether and stick to cooked forms only. You can balance out your meal with a vegetarian roll made with cucumber, asparagus or avocado, instead of fish. **Avocados** are an excellent source of heart-healthy, skin-enhancing monounsaturated fats, but they are also higher in calories than other vegetables, so don't go overboard with them. If fish is not your thing or you're vegetarian or vegan, you can opt for **tofu** or a side dish of **edamame**; both are excellent alternative sources of protein.

2. Go light on the rice The basic rolls, such as plain fish, avocado and cucumber, are all good choices, but they do come with white rice, which is high in calories and low in nutritional value. As it contains practically no fibre or protein, the calories quickly add up, and get converted straight into simple sugars and fat. That doesn't mean, however, that white rice can't be incorporated into a healthy diet in the right way. My advice is to try to get brown rice sushi, which is becoming more widely available in shops and restaurants, particularly in London, wherever possible. This will provide your body with added fibre, protein and various other nutrients, such as B vitamins, so that a smaller serving of sushi will get you satiated sooner, and for longer, as well as providing your body with added healthy nutrition.

If brown rice is not on offer, order sashimi – at least as the bulk of your meal – and perhaps have one vegetable roll made with rice on the side. Ordering sashimi will save you a lot in refined carbs and calories, and packs in a hefty dose of high-quality protein and essential omega-3 fatty acids.

3. Don't be tempted by tempura Stay away from anything on the menu labelled as 'crunchy' or 'tempura', as this indicates that the rolls or fish inside are coated in batter or breadcrumbs, and deep fried. Forgo the fat and extra calories by avoiding these dishes altogether.

4. Know your portions While traditional sushi is a healthy food it's still important to stick to proper portions if your aim is to eat light and stay slim. An average sushi roll (about six pieces) contains around 250 calories. Thus, if you consume three rolls, which is not difficult, this amounts to a lot of calories – even before taking any added sauces or side dishes into account. As a guide, a sensible sushi meal would consist of a portion of sashimi pieces (about six pieces) and one to two basic rolls – such as salmon, avocado, cucumber or corn, or two rolls (twelve pieces) of a bulkier variety.

5. Be mindful In the same vein, because sushi is cut into those little pieces that pop perfectly into your mouth, it makes every extra bite seem so harmless. It's definitely a moreish kind of food that's very easy to 'lose track' of. This is especially true if you're sharing rolls with family or friends, or eating them standing at an engagement party or wedding reception, as opposed to ordering a takeaway meal or dining in a restaurant. A good strategy is to put all the sushi you plan to eat on your plate *before* you tuck in, as this will prevent you getting carried away. Also, make use of those chopsticks – they'll force you to eat more slowly.

Greek

Greek food is one of the world's healthiest cuisines. Typical of the famed Mediterranean diet, it's full of heart-healthy mono-unsaturated fats (in olives and olive oil), fish and vegetables. Although there's plenty of goodness to be had when dining Greek-style, there are a few dishes that are diet disasters. *Pastitsio* (a pasta casserole with ground lamb topped with a creamy béchamel sauce) and moussaka are both filled with rich cream sauce, translating into a hefty amount of calories and fat. While phyllo dough might seem flaky and light, each layer is actually brushed with butter to make it crisp. For a waist-friendly approach, start with Greek salad (dressing on the side), then have a grilled Greek-cuisine classic, such as grilled fish with vegetables. An alternative good choice to start would be whole-wheat pitta with a few tablespoons of hummus, tzatziki (yoghurt cucumber dip) or *baba ghanoush* (aubergine dip); just make sure they're enjoyed in moderation.

Middle Eastern

There are plenty of healthy options on the menu in Middle-Eastern-style dining, but at the same time there is also plenty of room to go wrong. The breads and spreads are delicious, but they can pack in hundreds of unnecessary calories, so be careful.

The option of getting any meat or falafel served in a *laffa* (thick white bread) or pitta bread 'sandwich' with generous helpings of hummus and tahini, not to mention the trend of adding French fries to it, is far from waist friendly. Skip the *laffa* or pitta and you'll save hundreds of calories. In terms of your choice of protein, *shawarma* is the worst and should be avoided. It's usually lamb, which is a 'stay away' food in the tables (see page 25), and even if it is chicken, it's dripping in oil and fat, and has the skin included – definitely not what you want to be choosing for both health and weight reasons. A lamb or beef shish kebab (on a plate with salads, not in a pitta) is definitely better and less fatty, and can be eaten occasionally, once you're at the lifestyle phase and fancy it as a treat. But your best bet (which you could even enjoy during the attack phase) is any form of grilled chicken (ideally breast, but thigh is also OK as long as it doesn't have the skin on) on a platter with salads or vegetables. Make sure you stick to non-fried options of veggies and salads, pickled vegetables, carrot salad or shredded cabbage salad, rather than going for calorie-laden deep-fried aubergine.

Indian

Traditional Indian dishes that feature a variety of vegetables, chickpeas, beans, lentils and rice are great for a low-GI, high-fibre, healthy, plant-based way of eating – exactly what The Food Effect prescribes. Moreover, Indian cuisine often includes plenty of grilled chicken options for those who want some animal protein. Combining these with some tomato-based side dishes such as beans or chickpeas and vegetables in light (non-creamy) sauces makes the perfect meal in both the attack and lifestyle phases. Although The Food Effect approach advocates brown rice over white, Indian basmati rice is an exception (as explained in Chapter 3) – although white, basmati rice is higher in protein and fibre than regular white rice, so you can enjoy it guilt-free.

While Indian food and many of the curries can be healthy, there are definitely some things to avoid. Some curries are made with large amounts of full-fat coconut milk or cream, so don't be too shy to ask a waiter how the dish is prepared. Avoid samosas (deep-fried pastries filled with meat or vegetables), and if you choose to have some bread with your meal (you certainly can once you are on the lifestyle phase), stick with a small portion of baked breads such as naan or whole-wheat chapatti, and avoid any fried breads.

A Final word on dining out

Remember that there's not a restaurant out there that demands you finish what's put in front of you. Think about the amount of food you've been served, eat slowly, enjoy your food and don't be afraid to leave anything that seems excessive.

Healthy eating when travelling and at the airport

Whether you're taking off on a long-planned holiday, heading home or travelling for work, being 'on the road' can wreak havoc on the best-laid eating plans. Travellers are often faced with a dilemma: either bring your own food, which takes some planning and foresight, or buy a meal or snack on the way to or at the airport, which may result in limited selection and poor nutritional choices. Airports in particular can be a challenge – giant muffins, multipacks of chocolates and sweets, fast-food restaurants and temptation galore. But travelling needn't ruin your weight-loss efforts. Follow the tips below for eating healthily when travelling and on the go.

- **Snack sensibly** The processed snacks that are the mainstay of airport shops don't satisfy hunger for very long. Processed foods that are high in fat and refined sugar, such as crisps, biscuits and milk chocolate bars, are all digested very quickly, raise your blood-sugar levels rapidly, and actually promote hunger and cravings. Instead, go for nuts as they are naturally filling, extremely healthy and contribute to stable blood-sugar levels (preventing further hunger and cravings). Bags of nuts are a staple at airport shops and indeed are a healthy choice (refer to 'eat this' in the tables, page 23). Nuts are a great source of protein, fibre and heart-healthy fats, and a single 30g serving contains only about 130 calories. But beware of those jumbo-size bags that can contain a whopping ten servings and can easily add up to a whole day's worth of calories. Do your own portioning as single servings into small Ziploc bags or Tupperware containers to pack into your hand luggage when travelling.

  If this is impossible to do in advance, buy nuts in pre-portioned bags (30–50g) so you don't overeat. Alternatively, pack some home-made 'energy balls' (see recipes on page 241–242), either of which make the perfect, portable filling snack. They are quick and easy to make, and you can easily make a batch ahead of time and keep them in the freezer for when you'll be travelling or on the go.
- **Fresh fruit never fails** Fresh fruit and chopped vegetables with hummus make smart, filling, on-the-go snacks. Whole fresh fruit and ready-cut fruit salads are sold at many airport shops, or you can easily pack an apple or two in your bag.
- **Beware of hidden ingredients** Items that may seem healthy, for example a tuna or egg sandwich, are often loaded with full-fat mayonnaise and oil, packing in more than 20g of fat per

sandwich. What's more, these sandwiches come ready made, so you do not have the option of asking for them without the mayo. Read labels to check ingredients and calories, and stick to sandwiches on wholemeal bread with vegetables and lean protein, such as smoked salmon or chicken, with either little or low-fat mayonnaise.

• **Grab a coffee** If healthy food is nowhere in sight and your stomach is rumbling, grab a tall skimmed or soya milk latte. The milk is full of protein and calcium, and is extremely filling and satisfying, especially if paired with some fresh fruit such as an apple.

• **Stay hydrated** Dehydration can make you feel tired and hungry, when actually you're really just thirsty. In fact, dehydration, both on the ground and in the air, can mimic the symptoms of hunger and cause you to overeat, when all you really need is to drink. Water is nature's perfect thirst quencher and it's totally calorie-free. It also helps to keep your skin healthy and glowing, which is important, as travelling and plane journeys can do just the opposite.

*

As you can see from this chapter, awareness and a little thought are all that's needed to make healthy choices when dining out or travelling. No longer does being on a diet mean that you are stuck at home having to eat a salad every night. From day one on the Food Effect diet, you can enjoy eating out with family and friends, while sticking to the plan and losing weight.

CHAPTER 9

Raise Your Glass

Moderate alcohol consumption is part of the programme!

Now here's the part you've been waiting for – can you drink alcohol on The Food Effect diet? I have good news for you: the answer is yes, even from day one. During the first four weeks – the attack phase and therefore the strictest part of the diet – you are allowed up to three drinks per week. I discuss what that means and the best choices to make below. Once you have completed the first four weeks of the diet and are on to the lifestyle phase, you can have up to one drink (that is, one glass of alcohol) per evening (or the equivalent, seven drinks in total, per week).

While it is true to say that heavy drinking is indeed unhealthy, and is linked to heart and liver disease, as well as an increased risk of various cancers; moderate drinking, which is what The Food Effect diet allows, has been shown to be extremely beneficial for the heart and circulatory system, and may even protect against Type 2 diabetes. Moderate drinking, if done wisely, will not compromise your weight-loss goals either. There are numerous studies showing that moderate alcohol consumption reduces the risk of obesity and weight gain. One study that followed more than 19,000 women for a period of nearly thirteen years revealed that women who consumed 1–2 alcoholic beverages daily were at least 30 per cent less likely to gain weight than non-drinkers. In another 2004 study conducted at the Departments of Nutrition and Epidemiology, Harvard School of Public Health, researchers reported that one drink per day did not contribute to weight gain, especially in women. In fact, alcohol may increase metabolism slightly so that you actually burn more calories. Researchers have found that consuming alcohol after a meal increased the number of calories burnt after both high- and low-carbohydrate meals. This may help explain the finding of these researchers, and many others, that moderate drinkers have less body fat than abstainers.

More recently, research has increasingly suggested that moderate alcohol consumption does not represent a dietary risk factor for developing obesity. In fact, a study published in the *Archives of Internal Medicine* found that light to moderate drinkers gain less weight than teetotallers over time, and have a decreased chance of becoming overweight or obese. I've seen this myself, first-hand, with clients who consistently lose weight without abstaining from alcohol. In fact, a study from Finland that included a total of 24,604 randomly selected men and women aged 25–64 concluded that 'A physically active lifestyle with abstention from smoking, moderate alcohol consumption, and consumption of healthy foods maximises the chances of having a normal weight.'

As already mentioned, most diets are temporary and people only stick to them for a certain period of time because they are too restrictive; and most diets make you cut out alcohol completely as well. Many people enjoy a glass of wine with dinner, or a drink with friends when out at the weekend, or with colleagues on an evening out after work. This is something many of my clients told me when they first came to see me, so to tell them to cut out alcohol altogether was simply not realistic (or I could have done so, but they wouldn't have listened). On top of that, feeling deprived over a long period of time sets you up for failure far more than a 100-calorie glass of wine does.

I knew that if people were to truly embrace The Food Effect as a lifestyle, moderate alcohol consumption had to be part of the programme. That doesn't mean I shied away from advising people to cut back on their consumption – or that they always found it easy. When a busy trader, for example, came to see me looking to lose weight and get healthier, I advised him to cut down from three drinks after work every night, and even more at the weekend, to a maximum of one drink a night. It was a challenge, but if I'd told him alcohol was not allowed at all, he would simply have given up on The Food Effect diet altogether. Being teetotal simply wouldn't fit into the social aspect of his corporate lifestyle. Acknowledging this was an important factor that I kept in mind in creating The Food Effect diet, and it's another reason why it is so doable and successful.

To help you decide what to order at the bar without compromising your weight-loss goals, here is The Food Effect guide to alcohol (stick to the limits according to the two phases as specified above – three drinks per week during phase one; seven drinks per week in phase two).

DRINK THIS	BE CAREFUL	STAY AWAY
Bloody Mary	Beer	Alcopops
Champagne	Mimosa	Amaretto Sour
Gin/vodka and diet tonic	Pina colada	Cocktails mixed with energy drinks
Red/white wine spritzer	Rum and Diet Coke	Cocktails with cola mixers
Red wine	Vodka cranberry	Eggnog
Vodka and mineral water with lemon/lime		Frozen daiquiri
White wine		Malibu and Coke/fruit juice
		Margarita
		Milky/creamy liqueurs

As with everything on The Food Effect diet, the key is to make the right choices.

During the attack phase, make sure your three drinks per week come from the 'drink this' column in the above table. During the lifestyle phase, try to stick to the 'drink this' column, but if you occasionally choose a drink from the 'be careful' list, that's also perfectly fine. Just ensure you don't make those drinks your regular tipple (that is, what you choose every night).

Throughout the lifestyle phase, try to avoid all the 'stay away' drinks. Like the foods in the food tables listed in Chapter 2, they are in the 'stay away' column for a reason – they do nothing to benefit your overall health and weight-loss goals and should be avoided, or taken only on the very odd occasion.

Make sensible choices

Since you've now read that drinking in moderation is not unhealthy and will not cause weight gain (in fact, it may even help with weight loss), you know there's no need to give up alcohol. However, the key is to remain sensible and stick to the rules of 'moderation'.

The UK Chief Medical Officer's guidelines for both men and women are that to keep health risks from alcohol to a low level it is safest not to drink more than 14 units a week on a regular basis. The guidelines, which were updated in 2016, made the recommended limit the same for men as women. This equals 6 pints of average strength beer a week, which would mean a low risk of illnesses such as liver disease or cancer. The previous guidelines were 21 units for men and 14 units for women per week. An additional recommendation is not to 'save up' the 14 units for 1 or 2 days, but to spread them over 3 or more days. This is exactly in line with The Food Effect guidelines for both phases of the diet.

For The Food Effect diet I have also kept the rules the same for both men and women and allow three drinks per week during the four-week attack phase, and one drink per evening (or seven drinks per week) during the lifestyle phase.

One standard alcoholic drink is:

• One small bottle (330ml) of regular (5%) beer (1.6 units, 142 calories).
• 175ml glass of (13%) wine (2.3 units, 159 calories)
• A shot (25ml) of spirits (40%) such as vodka, tequila or rum, either straight or in a mixed drink (1 unit, 61 calories, not including sugary mixes/soft drinks/fruit juice).

You also have to be mindful, especially once you're on the life-style phase, that you cannot have alcohol *and* that little bit extra of a dark chocolate dessert, or an extra red meat steak for the week. It's all about making choices and deciding which option you will enjoy indulging in more – the alcohol or the food. If you're dining out and fancy pasta with tomato sauce (no cream) that night, you might want to lay off a second glass of red wine. If you're desperate to enjoy two glasses of alcohol one night, choose the fish and salad instead of the pizza or pasta.

Another thing to be cautious of is alcohol potentially put-ting you in an 'Oh, why not?' frame of mind, that results in you eating or drinking too much. If drinking alcohol lowers your inhibitions to the extent that you wind up gorging on the contents of the bread basket or the salted bar snacks, then plan ahead and either make sure you've had a filling, satisfying meal or snack before you go out for drinks, or if you're drinking while dining out, ask for a plate of vegetable crudités to snack on until your meal arrives – that dish of salted nuts can easily pack in several hundred calories before your meal even arrives. Also make sure you drink water between sips of alcohol to stay well hydrated and satisfied, and switch to water or sparkling water with lemon after you've had your one drink.

Remember why you enjoy having a drink in the first

place – that is, to enjoy the time with friends, family or colleagues, *not* so that you can overindulge. There's no reason why
alcohol should ever interfere with your healthy-eating choices.
You can have a great time, enjoy alcohol in moderation and
make The Food Effect diet work.

A few more tips

As you can see from the table above, your best bets for healthy
low-calorie drinks are wine and spirits. If mixed drinks are more
your thing, order less-caloric, lower sugar versions of your usual
drink. For example, order rum and Diet Coke instead of rum
and Coke. (While I'm no advocate of drinking Diet Coke just
for the sake of it, in this instance it's far better for your health
and weight than regular sugar-laden Coke.) Or order vodka,
tequila or other spirits with zero-calorie soda water and a splash
of cranberry juice, instead of a sugar-laden lemonade. Or have
a wine spritzer that is half wine, half soda water. Do beware of
sugary cocktails such as Margaritas, Long Island Iced Teas and
Pina Coladas, which can set you back anywhere from 400 to 650
calories – that's more than a Big Mac. Opt instead for tequila on
the rocks with a splash of lime cordial or juice, or vodka mixed
with soda water and cranberry juice.

If you're out at a special event or social situation where everyone is ordering cocktails at the bar, either stick to one of the
above if possible, or have just one cocktail, then switch to water
or sparkling water garnished with lemon or lime. I can assure
you no one will be any the wiser – you won't seem like a party
pooper, *and* you won't derail your health and weight-loss goals
either.

CHAPTER 10

Exercise and Supplements

Stop stressing about the gym – it's all about what you eat

Relying on exercise for weight loss is a major mistake that many people make because they've been led to believe it plays a big part in achieving great results. While keeping active definitely plays a part in a sustainable weight-loss regime, it is certainly not the *major* part in it. You can exercise all you like, but if you are eating a bad diet full of saturated fat, sugar and processed foods full of trans fats and additives – you are unlikely to see any results. As any personal trainer will tell you: 'Abs are made in the kitchen', and 'You can't out-train a bad diet.'

The scientific facts back this up. In the past thirty years as obesity has rocketed, there has been little change (that is, no significant decline) in physical activity levels in Western populations. This places the blame for our expanding waistlines solely on the type and amount of calories consumed.

There are many people out there who think that it is OK to eat a packet of biscuits, a big piece of cake or big slab of milk chocolate, because they will go for a run straight afterwards. This is no way to lose weight and achieve the results you want.

In fact, you're putting in all that effort for nothing. The key to weight loss is what goes in your mouth. If you feel like eating a piece of cake or a biscuit, go ahead and have one. But know that you've strayed from The Food Effect way of eating and might not lose weight that day. That's normal and OK (on the odd occasion). But don't get into the habit of eating badly and thinking you can exercise it off. It simply doesn't work and will leave you feeling dejected and upset at the lack of positive results.

While I definitely advocate *some* form of exercise (even if it's just walking) on most days, I don't encourage my clients or those adopting The Food Effect lifestyle to spend a huge amount of time on exercise, or to have an unhealthy focus on it, as it is not the key to (or even a large part of) weight loss. Weight loss requires patience, effort and dedication to eating well. Excess weight is not something you can simply 'run off' in the park. It may take a while (by that I mean several weeks, *not* years) but if done correctly, staying slim and in shape can be sustainable for your entire life. Don't make yourself miserable in pursuit of a quick fix by driving yourself crazy over exercise – it really isn't worth it and it doesn't work either.

In an editorial published in the *British Journal of Sports Medicine*, three leading international health experts said it was time to 'bust the myth' about exercise. They concluded that while physical activity was a key part of staving off diseases such as diabetes, heart disease and dementia, its impact on tackling obesity was minimal, hence public health messages should squarely focus on unhealthy eating rather than exercise. The experts also pointed to evidence from the *Lancet* global burden of disease programme, which shows that unhealthy eating was linked to more ill-health than physical inactivity, alcohol and smoking combined. They blamed the food industry, with its advertising and celebrity endorsements, for encouraging the belief that exercise could counteract the impact of unhealthy eating. 'An obese person does not need to do one iota of exercise to lose weight; they just need to eat less. My biggest concern is that the messaging that is coming to the public suggests you can eat what you like as long as you exercise,' said leading London cardiologist Dr Aseem Malhotra. 'That is unscientific and wrong. You cannot outrun a bad diet.'

The Food Effect approach is directly in line with what these experts recommend. Countless overweight clients have come to me, having been misinformed that if they want to lose weight they need to exercise intensely every day. They believed that in order to be slim, they had to 'kill themselves' at the gym or take up running. Many had been training rigorously with a personal trainer for months, getting up early for boot camps that they loathed, or spending almost every day in the gym (despite not enjoying it) for the sole purpose of losing weight, but the pounds had not shifted. These despondent, over-exercised clients all arrived at my practice overweight, frustrated and desperate – quite understandably.

On changing their diets (and, with many clients, even exercising less), the pounds dropped off. I had one client, who during our initial phone call before starting at The Food Effect clinic, told me, 'My biggest problem is that I don't have time to exercise, so I can't lose weight.' I reassured him that he didn't need to do an iota of exercise (I'm not saying that's the ideal for health, but weight-loss-wise it would make no difference), and if he changed the way he ate, he could lose weight. Sure enough, David never took on any exercise, followed The Food Effect programme and lost 42lb, reaching his goal weight in just six months.

Why exercise doesn't result in weight loss

Now that we've established that exercise isn't as useful for weight loss as you may have been led to believe, I'll briefly explain the science behind why this is.

1. **It increases appetite** While you may not feel hungry imme-
    diately after a workout, you'll definitely notice that on the
    days you've exercised your appetite increases later in the
    day. If you've ever been swimming or had an intense morn-
    ing workout, you'll have noticed that you get ravenous later
    in the day. Often, you end up eating more calories on those
    days than you actually burnt off, because your hunger is
    so much greater. On top of increased appetite, exercising
    makes your body crave high-calorie foods to replace the lost
    energy from intense workouts, making it that much more
    difficult to resist a post-workout binge.

2. **Exercise doesn't burn that many calories** Unfortunately,
    exercise doesn't burn as many calories as we'd like it to. It's
    much easier to resist a 300-calorie Mars bar, than to burn 300
    calories on a treadmill. Unless you're doing triathlon training,
    exercise will probably only burn around 10 per cent of your
    energy intake per day. When you consider that your appetite
    increases and that exercise makes you crave high-calorie
    foods, it's even harder to achieve any significant calorie deficit.

3. **We overestimate how hard we have trained** Because exercise
    can feel strenuous and exhausting, it's common to think
    you've burnt more calories than you have. People generally
    overestimate how many calories they've burnt, while under-
    estimating how much they eat.

4. **Our bodies adapt** The human body is highly intelligent.
    When you exercise a lot and often, your body becomes more
    efficient at storing calories, and you end up burning fewer of
    them. This is known as metabolic compensation.

5. **Exercise can increase cortisol and promote fat storage**
    Although exercise does increase metabolism, when you
    push yourself too much, it can have the opposite effect and
    prevent weight loss. Pushing ourselves to do long runs, for
    example, can cause the body to release the stress hormone
    cortisol to keep us going, yet this hormone also encourages
    fat storage around the middle.

6.   **We can begin to resent exercise** As I've witnessed first-hand through clients, when you think you need to exercise to lose weight and don't see the number on the scales dropping, you become resentful and begin to despise exercise. This can sabotage your relationship with physical activity, which should be something enjoyable and part of maintaining good health, not viewed as a chore and a punishment carried out solely in a misguided attempt to lose weight.

If exercise won't help with weight loss, why should you do it?

I've told you that exercise is not the key to weight loss, and described the science behind why this is the case. However, you do need to do *some* physical activity for the sake of your health. Here are some things it is certainly beneficial for. Exercise:

1.   **Boosts your mood** Exercise is proven to boost mood, and even to help counteract stress and anxiety and ward off depression. Exercise releases mood-boosting endorphins and helps release stress, making you feel noticeably happier after physical activity.

2.   **Helps concentration and makes you smarter** Even a short ten-minute workout (such as one taken from a YouTube video), or a brisk walk outdoors, will instantly boost your concentration and aid cognitive performance. One study even showed that exercise can make you smarter by helping to grow so many new brain cells (a process called neurogenesis) that your brain actually gets bigger.

3.   **Increases your lifespan** The same study outlined above revealed that exercise has a beneficial effect on your genes, helping to reverse the ageing process at a cellular level.

4. **Lowers your blood pressure**, thereby reducing the risk of heart attacks and stroke.
5. **Increases bone density**, reducing the risk of osteoporosis and fractures.
6. **Improves balance**, so that there is less risk of falls and fractures.
7. **Increases strength, flexibility and stamina.**
8. **Helps improve sleep.**
9. **Gives you more energy for both work and play.**

What sort of exercise should you do?

Exercise doesn't need to be complicated. To gain all the health benefits of exercise listed above, you don't have to join a gym, hire a personal trainer or sign up for a marathon. My advice is simply to do what you enjoy, make it as enjoyable as you can and do it regularly.

If you're currently not doing much exercise or any at all, try walking for at least 10–20 minutes every day (this can include walks to work, to the train, between public transport and so on). This is not only good for your bones, body and circulation, but it also gives you time to think, breathe and de-stress – all essential to a healthy lifestyle. Light exercise also helps to lower the stress hormones cortisol and adrenalin, high levels of which can be responsible for excess weight storage (especially abdominal fat, as explained earlier). On top of your light daily walking, try working out (anything that raises your heart rate) for either ten minutes 5–6 times a week, or twenty minutes three times a week – you don't have to kill yourself to become fit and toned. You'll notice a difference to how you look and feel simply by adopting that.

If you *do* already love to exercise, and are doing more than that – that's fantastic and I'm obviously not going to tell you to stop. A study in *Nutrition and Metabolism* showed that those who see exercise as part of their lifestyle, rather than as a way to change their appearance, are most successful at keeping the weight off.

Get supplement savvy

This is an important topic in the health and fitness world right now, and a subject that I'm always asked my advice and opinion about. That's hardly surprising given that the spectrum of supplements available today is so overwhelming. What should you take, and when? Ask some people and you'll get an endless list that would cost you a small fortune. Of course, some people with particular dietary restrictions or medical conditions require supplements, but most of us can get everything we need from a colourful, varied and balanced diet. If you follow The Food Effect meal options and plans, this is certainly the case. Vegetarians and vegans may benefit from taking vitamin B12 and omega-3, but if you eat fish, and/or even walnuts, supplementing with omega-3 is not necessary.

Don't be D-ficient
While I'm not one for advocating an array of supplements and vitamins (other than in the form of food), there is one vitamin that I've always advocated, and tell all my clients – men, women and children – to take, and that's vitamin D. This 'sunshine vitamin' has recently become the rising star of the supplement world (finally!) due to research suggesting that it does far more than protect against soft bones and rickets.

Low levels of this vitamin have been associated with increased fat storage, among many other health problems – and the sad reality for those of us living in the UK, is ▶

that we are definitely lacking in some good old sunshine. Levels of vitamin D deficiency in the UK are the highest in fifty years, with one in five people suffering severe deficiency. The incidence of infant rickets, the bone-weakening condition that was rife in Victorian slums, was at a record high in 2015. Experts have attributed the problem to indoor lifestyles, the increased use of sunscreen, poor diet and cool summers.

While vitamin D may be best known for promoting healthy bone growth, in fact most organs require (and therefore have receptors for) vitamin D. We now know that low levels (which are virtually guaranteed in everyone during the winter in the UK), are associated with an increased risk of conditions ranging from heart disease, multiple sclerosis and Alzheimer's disease, to diabetes, breast cancer and bowel cancer. Even a mild to moderate deficiency can, in the long term, result in osteoporosis, making fractures more likely in a fall.

Additionally, as mentioned above, vitamin D levels have an impact on weight. Vitamin D deficiency causes the brain to issue hunger-signalling hormones, tempting you to reach for the biscuit tin. Calcium-rich diets have also been found to aid weight loss, but vitamin D is required to regulate calcium absorption. Therefore you should definitely take a vitamin D supplement from October to March, if not all year round. Most of us have a deficiency of vitamin D in the summer as well, so keeping our levels up in the winter is crucial.

Although vitamin D is found in foods such as oily fish, eggs (the yolks) and fortified cereals, it's virtually impossible to consume enough of these to get an adequate amount through diet alone. You'd need to consume ten eggs (yolks included) to reach the required 10mcg per day.

The body depends mainly on internal production through the action of sunlight on the skin – which unfortunately we do not get enough of in the UK. Even if you live in a hot country, unless you sit out and sunbathe daily, it's unlikely that you will get enough of this vitamin through sunlight alone.

UK guidelines previously only recommended routine supplementation for those most at risk of deficiency (the elderly, pregnant and breastfeeding women, and so on). However, my advice to all would be to take a standard dose vitamin D supplement – which can be found in chemists and health-food stores – every day (1,000 IU per day). Thankfully, new national guidelines from Public Health England are now in line with what I recommend at The Food Effect clinic; as of 2016 their advice is that all Britons should consider taking a daily supplement of vitamin D, particularly from October to March. Doctors (myself included) welcomed this guidance, saying that vitamin D deficiency could be eliminated entirely with supplements costing an average of just £10 to £15 a year.

A few final words on exercise and tips to get you started

After reading this chapter, hopefully you'll understand why exercise is not the key to weight loss, and that the main factor in losing weight and staying slim is what goes in your mouth.

However, there are far too many health and lifestyle benefits from exercise not to make it part of your routine. Here are some tips to help you as you begin The Food Effect diet and way of life.

- Check with your doctor first. If you are severely overweight or have any serious medical conditions, it is advisable to get your doctor's approval before embarking on an exercise programme.
- Choose activities that you enjoy. If you're having fun and enjoying yourself, even if you're working hard, you're more likely to stick to a routine.
- Set aside a regular time for exercise. Whether you sign up to an exercise class or decide to wake up a little earlier every day to do some exercise, scheduling it in as you would a work meeting will guarantee that nothing gets in the way of your good intentions.
- Partner up with a friend, family member or your partner. This makes it more fun and will increase motivation and commitment to your new fitness regime.
- Vary your exercise. There is no 'best' or 'right' exercise, just what works best for you. It's never easy, especially at the start, but once you begin to feel better, and have more energy and a new zest for life, you'll never want to give it up.

CHAPTER 11

Phase 1, Kickstart Your Weight Loss

The Food Effect attack phase and meal options

This phase is all about kickstarting your weight loss and helping to banish cravings for good. It's the strictest phase of the diet, but you'll still be eating plenty (including carbs and dark chocolate). It lasts for four weeks – just twenty-eight days – which is long enough to completely resolve any insulin resistance brought about by eating too many unhealthy, processed carbs and foods. During this phase you will be completely red-meat free – so while you'll still be allowed chicken, fish, dairy foods and eggs, you should avoid lamb, beef or pork. Keeping to this plan for four weeks gives meat eaters a chance to explore other protein options. You'll see that there really is no hardship in sacrificing a steak for some vegetable, chicken or fish options. Once you move on to The Food Effect lifestyle phase, you'll be allowed red meat once a week, if you still want it.

Phase one is *not* low carb – it's about eating the right amount of the right carbs. You aren't, however, allowed things like whole-wheat pasta or breakfast cereals during this phase, but you can reintroduce them once you reach The Food Effect lifestyle phase.

The meal plan is designed to allow ample portions of healthy protein, good fats, vegetables and low-GI carbs, needed for optimum satisfaction and blood-sugar stability. This includes low-GI fruit (such as apples, pears and berries) and starchy vegetables (such as sweet potato), where portions are specified. There is no benefit in cutting these out – they contribute fibre, important nutrients, vitamins and minerals, and heart-healthy antioxidants. Most salads and vegetables (including all green vegetables, carrots, tomatoes, cauliflower and butternut) are unlimited. The proteins come from a wide range of sources, ranging from poultry to plant-based proteins, so you can be flexible. If you're vegetarian or don't eat eggs, for example, you can substitute them with another specified protein source. By the time this phase ends, any unhealthy cravings you have for sweets, chocolate, baked goods and unhealthy starches will essentially have vanished. Even though this is the strictest phase, you will by no means be going hungry. You'll be eating three substantial meals, plus two satisfying snacks (including a post-dinner/late-evening treat) a day, so you'll certainly never feel deprived.

The meal plan is laid out day by day for ease and simplicity, but you can interchange any of the options within the same meal category on any given day – that is, switch the specified breakfast for any of the breakfasts from any of the days, and the same for lunches and dinners. You can't interchange a lunch for a dinner, for example; you can only interchange meals and snacks that are within the same categories. In short, as long as you consume *no more* than a specified breakfast, lunch, dinner and two snacks on each given day for twenty-eight days, you'll lose weight (around 6–12lb in the first four weeks alone, though as previously mentioned, this will depend on how much weight you have to lose, because the more excess weight you're carrying, the more you can expect to lose).

Keep moving (light activity, as long as you're not sedentary) each day, and don't forget to keep to The Food Effect principles and rules laid out in in Chapter 3 throughout the four weeks of this phase. As well as adhering to these rules, keep to the following few additional rules specific to the attack phase.

1. There should be no interchanging of meals between different categories (as explained above).

2. Make sure you have a glass of water with either a tablespoon of lemon juice or apple cider vinegar soon after waking every day (stevia or xylitol can be added to sweeten the drink). This will kickstart your metabolism and digestive system ready for the day ahead.

3. The only fruit allowed during this phase are apples, oranges, pears, grapefruit and berries. Occasionally, a small portion of dried fruit (such as raisins) is specified. (Once you move on to the lifestyle phase, all fruits are allowed, apart from bananas.)

4. Keep to a maximum of two slices of wholemeal or rye bread per day during this phase. Each day has already been designed this way for you – for example, if lunch is a sandwich, there won't be an option that includes a slice of toast for breakfast, so you don't have to think about this if you are following the specified meals. But if you do choose to interchange meals, make sure you do not exceed two slices of bread across all meals per day.

5. The carbohydrates to stick to that are included in the twenty-eight-day plan are minimally processed unrefined carbs – oats, quinoa, sweet potato, brown rice, wholemeal bread, Ryvita crackers, brown rice cakes and oatcakes. There is no whole-wheat pasta or whole-grain breakfast cereal in this phase – these are introduced into the meal options for the lifestyle phase.

6. Salads can be dressed and seasoned with lemon juice, balsamic vinegar or apple cider vinegar, plus herbs, salt and pepper. No olive oil should be added to salads (unless specified in a given recipe), and definitely no rich sauces or creamy dressings.

7. Drink at least 2 litres of water a day.
8. You can have two coffees or teas with skimmed or almond milk per day; all other hot drinks should be herbal teas.
9. You must have your mid-afternoon snack. Evening snacks are optional – many of my clients find they don't need them (or only have them on the odd night). You're certainly allowed these, but if you don't feel hungry, don't feel you must have them.
10. No mid-morning snacks – have a hot drink or herbal tea if you're peckish.
11. No 'cheat meals' during the attack phase. (The lifestyle phase does, however, allow room for indulgences, and being lenient on special occasions.)
12. No red meat *at all* during the attack phase. (This is reintroduced in moderation in the lifestyle phase.)
13. Weigh yourself every morning (without clothes on) during these twenty-eight days. As explained in the general rules, once you move on to the lifestyle phase, you'll only be expected to weigh yourself once a week.

A study in *The Journal of the Academy of Nutrition and Dietetics* found that weighing yourself every day leads to greater adoption of weight-control behaviours, and produces greater weight loss compared with weighing yourself most days of the week. The study showed that the more frequently people weighed themselves, the more 'cognitive restraint' they had for consuming unhealthy, fatty foods. In other words, you'll be less likely to grab a handful of greasy chips or a chocolate bar at work if you know it's going to make the scales go in the wrong direction. This is especially helpful to 'get you going' in the first four weeks of The Food Effect diet, which are the strictest, and occur when you're just beginning to cut out all the bad stuff and change your eating habits for the good.

You need as much discipline during this time as possible, and knowing that you have to step on the scales every morning definitely helps. Another added benefit of this is that it gives real encouragement to keep going as you see the number on the scales going down.

That being said, however, it's unrealistic to expect to see a drop every single day, so don't get despondent or expect this to happen – your weight may stay the same for several days, then you'll see a sudden drop. Also, things like sodium intake or, for women, having periods, can cause the body to retain more fluid and thus nudge up the number on the scales for a day or two. Don't worry – as long as you stick to your plan and keep going, you'll see the overall number drop by the end of the four weeks.

Once you've finished the attack phase, I recommend that you weigh yourself once a week (again first thing in the morning without clothes on) when you're on to The Food Effect lifestyle phase. Weekly monitoring will allow you to catch small weight gains, and initiate corrective behavioural and dietary changes, without obsessing about your weight.

Despite these additional rules, once you get started you'll be surprised at how doable it all is.

The twenty-eight day attack phase meal plan

Day 1

Breakfast
Perfect Porridge (see recipe page 192)
Served with 75g blueberries or mixed berries
Coffee or tea with skimmed or almond milk; or herbal tea

Lunch
Smoked Salmon and Avocado Salad:
2 slices smoked salmon (60g), plus ½ avocado (cubed or sliced)
Mixed salad (lettuce or spinach leaves, cherry tomatoes, cucumber, grated carrot, red or yellow pepper), tossed with balsamic or apple cider vinegar or lemon juice, salt and pepper
3 Ryvita crackers or brown rice cakes, or 1 slice wholemeal or rye toast

Afternoon snack
1 apple or pear, plus 2 oatcakes
Mug of herbal tea

Dinner
Quinoa Salad with Roasted Vegetables
(see recipe page 203) – save half for lunch tomorrow
Served with mixed green salad and balsamic vinegar

Evening snack
30g dark chocolate (70 per cent cocoa or above)
and fruit (such as 1 apple, pear or orange)
Herbal tea

Day 2

Breakfast
Eggs with Greens:
Scramble or poach 2 eggs and serve with unlimited
spinach/rocket/steamed green beans
Coffee or tea with skimmed or almond milk; or herbal tea

Lunch
Quinoa Salad with Roasted Vegetables
(left over from last night's supper)
1 large apple

Afternoon snack
2 sticks of celery topped with 2 tbsp low-fat cottage cheese
Mug of herbal tea

Dinner
Chinese Chicken Stir-fry (see recipe page 211)
Served with 125g cooked brown rice
Mixed green salad drizzled with balsamic vinegar

Evening snack
Fresh fruit (apple, pear or orange), plus 15 almonds
Herbal tea

Day 3

Breakfast
1 slice wholemeal toast or 3 Ryvita
120g low-fat cottage cheese
150g strawberries or mixed berries
Coffee or tea with skimmed or almond milk; or herbal tea

Lunch
Mediterranean Salad (see recipe page 204)

Afternoon snack
1 orange and 12 almonds
Mug of herbal tea

Dinner
Spicy Stuffed Sweet Potato (see recipe page 206)
Mixed green salad, drizzled with balsamic vinegar

Evening snack
Baked Apple with Pecans:
1 baked apple (or fresh if preferred), sprinkled
with stevia, cinnamon and 2 tbsp chopped pecan nuts
Herbal tea

Day 4

Breakfast
Avocado Toast (see recipe page 193)
Served with fresh sliced tomato, seasoned
with salt and pepper
Coffee, tea or herbal tea

Lunch
Quinoa Tuna Salad:
185g cooked quinoa
½ tin of tuna (60g) (in water or brine)
Mixed salad (diced cucumber, tomato, red pepper)
1 tbsp low-fat mayonnaise, plus lemon juice,
salt and pepper

Afternoon snack
1 apple, plus 12 unsalted almonds or cashew nuts
Mug of herbal tea

Dinner
Spicy Tomato and Pepper Frittata (see recipe page 205) –
save half for tomorrow's lunch
Served with large mixed green salad,
plus balsamic vinegar

Evening snack
1 low-fat natural yoghurt (150g), plus 75g blueberries
Herbal tea

Day 5

Breakfast
Smoked Salmon on Toast:
1 slice wholemeal or rye bread, toasted
60g smoked salmon
Sliced cucumber or tomato, seasoned
with salt and pepper
1 pear
Coffee, tea or herbal tea

Lunch
Spicy Tomato and Pepper Frittata
(left over from last night's dinner)
Served with mixed green salad and balsamic vinegar

Afternoon snack
2 oatcakes, plus 2 tbsp reduced-fat hummus
Mug of herbal tea

Dinner
Avocado and Cottage Cheese Salad (see recipe page 207)

Evening snack
30g dark chocolate (70 per cent cocoa or above),
plus fruit (such as 1 apple, pear or orange)
Herbal tea

Day 6

Breakfast
Perfect Porridge (see recipe page 192)
Served with 1 tbsp mixed seeds (such as sunflower
seeds, pumpkin seeds or linseeds)
Coffee, tea or herbal tea

Lunch
Mackerel Salad:
1 tin (125g) of mackerel in tomato sauce
Mixed salad/spinach leaves
½ red pepper, sliced, chopped cucumber and 1 chopped tomato
Seasoned with lemon juice, salt and pepper

Afternoon snack
2 Ryvita or brown rice cakes, plus 2 tbsp low-fat cottage cheese
Mug of herbal tea

Dinner
Honey-roasted Chicken:
1 chicken breast (150g), drizzled with 1 tbsp honey
and soya sauce, grilled
Served with unlimited steamed broccoli and/or cauliflower
or Miraculous Cauliflower Mash (see recipe page 224)

Evening snack
Fresh fruit (apple, pear or orange), plus 15 almonds
Herbal tea

Day 7

Breakfast
1 boiled or poached egg
1 slice wholemeal bread, toasted
1 orange or ½ grapefruit (top with stevia or xylitol)
Coffee, tea or herbal tea

Lunch
Avocado, Spinach and Strawberry Salad
with Sweet Poppy Seed Dressing (see recipe page 208)

Afternoon snack
2 oatcakes, plus 2 tbsp reduced-fat hummus
Mug of herbal tea

Dinner
Baked Sweet Potato with Beetroot and Cottage Cheese
(see recipe page 209)

Evening snack
25g mixed dried fruit and nuts
Herbal tea

Day 8

Breakfast
170g 0% Greek yoghurt, with stevia (optional)
75g mixed berries (blueberries, blackberries and strawberries)
Drizzle of agave syrup (1 tsp)
Coffee, tea or herbal tea

Lunch
Smoked Salmon Sandwich on Rye:
Spread 2 slices rye bread with mustard,
add 2 slices smoked salmon, plus a handful of
fresh spinach leaves, and lemon juice, salt and pepper
Pre-cut carrot sticks on the side (unlimited)

Afternoon snack
1 apple plus 1 handful (12) almonds
Mug of herbal tea

Dinner
Avocado, Spinach and Strawberry Salad
with Sweet Poppy Seed Dressing (see recipe page 208)
Served with 60g smoked salmon

Evening snack
2 oatcakes or Ryvita crackers, plus 2 tbsp reduced-fat hummus
Herbal tea

Day 9

Breakfast
Smoked Salmon Omelette (see recipe page 194)
Served with fresh sliced tomatoes, seasoned
with salt and pepper
Coffee, tea or herbal tea

Lunch
Roasted Vegetable and Chickpea Salad (see recipe page 205)

Afternoon snack
1 orange, plus 12 unsalted cashew nuts
Mug of herbal tea

Dinner
Easy Roast Supper:
150g rotisserie chicken breast
Roasted vegetables (such as courgettes, mushrooms, red
peppers and red onions), cooked with minimal oil or spray oil,
and seasoned with herbs, garlic powder, salt and pepper
1 small baked sweet potato (150g) or Miraculous Butternut
Squash Mash (see recipe page 225)

Evening snack
30g dark chocolate (70 per cent cocoa or above),
plus fruit (such as 1 apple or pear)
Herbal tea

Day 10

Breakfast
Avocado Toast (see recipe page 193)
Served with fresh sliced tomato, seasoned with salt and pepper
Coffee, tea or herbal tea

Lunch
Quinoa Tuna Salad:
185g cooked quinoa
½ tin of tuna (60g) (in water or brine)
Mixed salad (diced cucumber, tomato, red pepper)
1 tbsp low-fat mayo plus lemon juice, salt and pepper

Afternoon snack
1 pear, plus 2 oatcakes
Mug of herbal tea

Dinner
Spicy Stuffed Sweet Potato (see recipe page 206)
Mixed green salad, drizzled with balsamic vinegar

Evening snack
Fresh fruit (apple, pear or orange), plus 15 almonds
Herbal tea

Day 11

Breakfast
Perfect Porridge (see recipe page 192)
Served with 1 mini-box (14g) or 2 tbsp raisins
Coffee, tea or herbal tea

Lunch
Smoked Salmon and Avocado Salad:
2 slices smoked salmon (60g), plus ½ avocado (cubed/sliced)
Mixed salad (lettuce/spinach leaves, cherry tomatoes,
cucumber, grated carrot, red/yellow pepper), tossed with
balsamic or apple cider vinegar or lemon juice, salt and pepper
3 Ryvita crackers or brown rice cakes,
or 1 slice wholemeal or rye toast

Afternoon snack
150g low-fat natural yoghurt, plus 75g blueberries
with stevia and cinnamon
Mug of herbal tea

Dinner
Spicy Tomato and Pepper Frittata (see recipe page 205) –
save half for tomorrow's lunch
Served with large mixed green salad, plus balsamic vinegar

Evening snack
Pear with Pecans:
Serve half a baked pear (or fresh if preferred),
sprinkled with stevia and cinnamon,
and 1 tbsp crushed pecan nuts
Herbal tea

Day 12

Breakfast
150g low-fat natural yoghurt
Served with 75g mixed berries,
plus 1 tablespoon pumpkin/sunflower seeds
Drizzle of agave syrup (1 tsp) with cinnamon
Coffee, tea or herbal tea

Lunch
Spicy Tomato and Pepper Frittata
(left over from last night's dinner)
Served with mixed green salad, drizzled with balsamic vinegar

Afternoon snack
2 oatcakes, plus 2 tbsp reduced-fat hummus
Mug of herbal tea

Dinner
Teriyaki Salmon:
Marinate 1 fillet of salmon (180g) in 3 tbsp soy sauce,
1 tsp olive oil, 1 tsp finely grated ginger and 1 tsp honey or
agave syrup. Preheat oven to 200°C/Gas 6. Place the salmon,
coated in marinade, on a baking tray lined with foil and bake
in oven for 10–12 minutes until cooked through.
Serve with unlimited mixed stir-fried
or roasted vegetables (in minimal oil/spray oil)

Evening snack
25g mixed dried fruit and nuts
Herbal tea

Day 13

Breakfast
1 boiled or poached egg
1 slice wholemeal bread, toasted
2 grilled tomato halves or fresh sliced tomato,
seasoned with salt and pepper
Coffee, tea or herbal tea

Lunch
Chicken or salmon salad:
Combine 150g cooked (grilled) chicken breast or
salmon fillet, unlimited mixed salad greens, 10 cherry
tomatoes and 1 sliced spring onion
Top with balsamic vinegar, plus herbs, salt and black pepper
On the side: 1 apple or pear

Afternoon snack
2 sticks of celery, topped with 2 tbsp low-fat cottage cheese
Mug of herbal tea

Dinner
Quinoa Salad with Roasted Vegetables (see recipe page 203) –
save half for lunch tomorrow
Served with mixed green salad, drizzled with balsamic vinegar

Evening snack
30g dark chocolate (70 per cent cocoa or above),
plus 150g strawberries or mixed berries
Herbal tea

Day 14

Breakfast
Coconut French Toast (see recipe page 194)
Served with 75g sliced strawberries
Coffee, tea or herbal tea

Lunch
Quinoa Salad with Roasted Vegetables
(left over from last night's dinner)
1 large apple

Afternoon snack
1 orange, plus 12 almonds
Mug of herbal tea

Dinner
Spicy Stuffed Sweet Potato (see recipe page 206)
Mixed green salad, drizzled with balsamic vinegar

Evening snack
Strawberries with Pecans:
75g sliced strawberries, plus 1 tbsp crushed pecan nuts,
mixed with stevia or xylitol
Herbal tea

Day 15

Breakfast
150g low-fat natural yoghurt
Served with 75g mixed berries,
plus 1 tbsp pumpkin/sunflower seeds
Drizzle of agave syrup (1 tsp)
Coffee, tea or herbal tea

Lunch
Mediterranean Salad (see recipe page 204)

Afternoon snack
2 oatcakes, plus 1 tbsp peanut butter
Mug of herbal tea

Dinner
150g grilled or baked chicken breast or
roasted chicken thigh (no skin)
Fresh spinach/salad greens
(drizzled with balsamic vinegar)
Diced fresh tomatoes or red pepper, seasoned
with salt and pepper
125g cooked quinoa or brown rice

Evening snack
30g dark chocolate (70 per cent cocoa or above),
plus fruit (such as 1 apple, pear or orange)
Herbal tea

Day 16

Breakfast
Smoked Salmon Omelette (see recipe page 194)
Served with 150g sliced strawberries
Coffee, tea or herbal tea

Lunch
Quinoa, Feta and Avocado Salad:
185g cooked quinoa
60g reduced-fat feta cheese
Diced cucumber, tomato and red pepper, plus ¼ avocado
Seasoned with lemon juice, salt and pepper

Afternoon snack
1 apple, plus 2 Ryvita or oatcakes
Mug of herbal tea

Dinner
Chicken, Spinach and Strawberry Salad
with Sweet Poppy Seed Dressing (see recipe page 207)

Evening snack
25g mixed dried fruit and nuts
Herbal tea

Day 17

Breakfast
Perfect Porridge (see recipe page 192)
Served with 75g blueberries
Coffee, tea or herbal tea

Lunch
The Food Effect Greek Salad (see recipe page 209)

Afternoon snack
1 apple or orange, plus 12 almonds
Mug of herbal tea

Dinner
Chinese Chicken Stir-fry (see recipe page 211)
Served with 125g cooked brown rice
Mixed green salad drizzled with balsamic vinegar

Evening snack
30g dark chocolate (70 per cent cocoa or above),
plus fruit (such as 1 apple, pear or orange)
Herbal tea

Day 18

Breakfast
Quick and Easy Vegetable Omelette or Scramble
(see recipe page 195)
3 Ryvita crackers or 1 slice wholemeal toast
Coffee, tea or herbal tea

Lunch
Roasted Vegetable and Chickpea Salad (see recipe page 205)

Afternoon snack
1 pear, plus 12 cashew nuts
Mug of herbal tea

Dinner
Teriyaki Salmon:
Marinate 1 fillet of salmon (180g) in 3 tbsp soya sauce, 1 tsp
olive oil, 1 tsp finely grated ginger and 1 tsp honey or agave
syrup. Preheat oven to 200°C/Gas 6. Place the salmon, coated
in marinade, on a baking tray lined with foil and bake
in oven for 10–12 minutes until cooked through.
Serve with unlimited mixed stir-fried or
roasted vegetables (in minimal oil/spray oil)

Evening snack
150g low-fat natural yoghurt,
plus 75g blueberries and stevia (optional)
Herbal tea

Day 19

Breakfast
170g 0% Greek yoghurt, sweetened with stevia and cinnamon
75g mixed berries (blueberries, blackberries, strawberries)
Drizzle of agave syrup (1 tsp)
Coffee, tea or herbal tea

Lunch
The Food Effect Skinny Chicken Salad Deluxe
(see recipe page 210)
Chicken may be substituted with 1 tin of tuna
(120g) in water or brine, if preferred

Afternoon snack
2 dried figs, plus 1 tbsp pumpkin seeds
Mug of herbal tea

Dinner
Quick and Easy Vegetable Omelette or Scramble
(see recipe page 195)
3 Ryvita crackers or 1 slice wholemeal toast

Evening snack
Baked Apple with Pecans:
1 baked apple (or fresh if preferred), sprinkled
with stevia, cinnamon and 2 tbsp chopped pecan nuts
Herbal tea

Day 20

Breakfast
Avocado Toast (see recipe page 193)
Served with fresh sliced tomato, seasoned with salt and pepper
Coffee, tea or herbal tea

Lunch
The Food Effect Greek Salad (see recipe page 209)

Afternoon snack
150g low-fat natural yoghurt, plus 75g blueberries
with stevia and cinnamon
Mug of herbal tea

Dinner
Turkey-stuffed Peppers (see recipe page 212)

Evening snack
Fresh fruit (apple, pear or orange), plus 15 almonds
Herbal tea

Day 21

Breakfast
1 slice wholemeal toast or 3 Ryvita
120g low-fat cottage cheese
Sliced fresh tomato, seasoned with herbs, salt and pepper
Coffee, tea or herbal tea

Lunch
Mixed Bean Salad:
Combine 1 small tin (150g) or ½ regular tin of mixed bean
salad, 1 red pepper, diced and unlimited mixed salad leaves
Drizzle with balsamic vinegar, plus herbs,
salt and black pepper
On the side: 1 apple or pear

Afternoon snack
2 oatcakes, plus 2 tbsp reduced-fat hummus
Mug of herbal tea

Dinner
Smoked Salmon Omelette (see recipe page 194)
Served with fresh salad greens (unlimited)

Evening snack
30g dark chocolate (70 per cent cocoa or above), plus 1 orange
Herbal tea

Day 22

Breakfast
Perfect Porridge (see recipe page 192)
Served with 1 tbsp mixed seeds
Coffee, tea or herbal tea

Lunch
Smoked Salmon Sandwich on Rye:
Spread 2 slices rye bread with mustard,
and add 2 slices smoked salmon, plus a handful of
fresh spinach leaves, and lemon juice, salt and pepper
Pre-cut carrot sticks – on the side (unlimited)

Afternoon snack
1 apple, plus 12 almonds
Mug of herbal tea

Dinner
Quinoa Salad with Roasted Vegetables
(see recipe page 203) – save half for lunch tomorrow
Served with mixed green salad drizzled with balsamic vinegar

Evening snack
150g low-fat natural yoghurt, plus 150g strawberries
with stevia and cinnamon
Herbal tea

Day 23

Breakfast
1 boiled or poached egg
1 slice wholemeal bread, toasted
2 grilled tomato halves or fresh sliced tomato,
seasoned with salt and pepper
Coffee, tea or herbal tea

Lunch
Quinoa Salad with Roasted Vegetables
(left over from last night's dinner)
1 large apple

Afternoon snack
Pre-cut carrot sticks, plus 2 tbsp reduced-fat hummus
Mug of herbal tea

Dinner
Baked Sweet Potato with Beetroot
and Cottage Cheese (see recipe page 209)

Evening snack
25g mixed dried fruit and nuts
Herbal tea

Day 24

Breakfast
1 slice wholemeal toast or 3 Ryvita crackers
120g low-fat cottage cheese
150g mixed berries
Coffee, tea or herbal tea

Lunch
Avocado, Spinach and Strawberry Salad
with Sweet Poppy Seed Dressing (see recipe page 208)

Afternoon snack
2 oatcakes, plus 2 tbsp reduced-fat hummus
Mug of herbal tea

Dinner
Smoked Salmon Omelette (see recipe page 194)
Served with fresh salad greens (unlimited)

Evening snack
30g dark chocolate (70 per cent cocoa or above),
plus fruit (such as 1 apple, pear or orange)
Herbal tea

Day 25

Breakfast
Avocado Toast (see recipe page 193)
Served with fresh sliced tomato, seasoned with salt and pepper
Coffee, tea or herbal tea

Lunch
Tuna and Sweetcorn Salad:
½ tin of tuna (60g) (in water or brine), mixed
with 1 tbsp low-fat mayonnaise
150g tinned sweetcorn
Mixed salad/vegetables (lettuce/spinach leaves, cucumber,
cherry tomatoes, grated carrot, red/yellow pepper), tossed with
balsamic vinegar or lemon juice, salt and pepper

Afternoon snack
150g low-fat natural yoghurt,
plus 150g strawberries with stevia and cinnamon
Mug of herbal tea

Dinner
Chinese Chicken Stir-fry (see recipe page 211)
Served with 125g cooked brown rice
Mixed green salad drizzled with balsamic vinegar

Evening snack
Baked Apple with Pecans:
1 baked apple (or fresh if preferred), sprinkled with stevia
and cinnamon, and 2 tbsp chopped pecan nuts
Herbal tea

Day 26

Breakfast
Perfect Porridge (see recipe page 192)
Served with 1 tbsp mixed seeds
(such as sunflower and pumpkin seeds)
Coffee, tea or herbal tea

Lunch
Cottage Cheese Salad:
120g low-fat cottage cheese
Mixed salad/vegetables (lettuce/spinach leaves, tomatoes,
cucumber, grated carrot, red/yellow pepper), seasoned with
balsamic vinegar or lemon juice, salt and pepper
3 Ryvita crackers or brown rice cakes,
or 1 slice wholemeal toast

Afternoon snack
150g strawberries, plus 12 almonds
Mug of herbal tea

Dinner
Smoked Salmon Omelette (see recipe page 194)
Served with large mixed green salad
dressed with balsamic vinegar

Evening snack
30g dark chocolate (70 per cent cocoa or above),
plus 1 apple or pear
Herbal tea

Day 27

Breakfast
1 slice wholemeal or rye bread (toasted)
60g smoked salmon
Sliced cucumber/tomato, seasoned with
lemon juice, salt and pepper
1 pear
Coffee, tea or herbal tea

Lunch
Mediterranean Salad (see recipe page 204)

Afternoon snack
2 oatcakes, plus 2 tbsp reduced-fat hummus
Mug of herbal tea

Dinner
Honey-roasted chicken:
1 chicken breast (150g)
topped with 1 tbsp honey and soya sauce, and grilled
Served with unlimited steamed broccoli and/or cauliflower
or Miraculous Cauliflower Mash (see recipe page 224)

Evening snack
Fresh fruit (apple, pear or orange), plus 15 almonds
Herbal tea

Day 28

Breakfast
Coconut French Toast (see recipe page 194)
Served with 75g sliced strawberries
Coffee, tea or herbal tea

Lunch
Mixed Bean Salad:
Combine 1 small or ½ regular tin of mixed bean salad (150g),
2 chopped tomatoes and unlimited mixed salad leaves
Drizzle with balsamic vinegar,
and sprinkle with herbs, salt and black pepper
Serve with 3 Ryvita crackers or brown rice cakes

Afternoon snack
1 apple, plus 1 handful (12) almonds
Mug of herbal tea

Dinner
Avocado and Cottage Cheese Salad (see recipe page 207)

Evening snack
30g dark chocolate (70 per cent cocoa or above),
plus 150g strawberries
Herbal tea

CHAPTER 12

Phase 2, Continued Weight Loss and Maintenance

The Food Effect lifestyle and meal options

After four weeks on phase one, you'll switch to the more liberal version of the 'diet' and start living The Food Effect lifestyle. You'll reintroduce even more healthy carbs, including whole-wheat pasta and low-sugar, whole-grain cereals. The weight loss will slow slightly from phase one, but should still be around 1–2lb per week until you reach your goal weight. At this point, this way of eating will have become a way of life – your regular healthy lifestyle, rather than a 'weight-loss programme'. You'll be knowledgeable enough about how The Food Effect diet works to enjoy all the flexibility of the plan, while staying slim and enjoying your food.

To follow The Food Effect lifestyle, simply choose any one breakfast, lunch, mid-afternoon snack, supper and evening snack per day to make up your day's worth of eating. Obviously you can eat less than this (for example if you don't feel you need or want an evening snack after dinner every day or want fewer crackers than specified with lunch), but you cannot have more than this per day. This way, you'll never exceed a calorie cap to make you gain weight or prevent you from losing it.

Unlike during the attack phase, you're now allowed more than two pieces of any wholemeal bread per day (as long as it fits into the meal options). So, for example, you can choose a breakfast option that includes a piece of toast, and lunch may be a sandwich. This doesn't mean that you should *aim* to do this every day, as variety is always good – but you are certainly allowed to do so, and it won't compromise your weight as long as you keep to the portions specified in the options.

There may be times once you're on the lifestyle, during your continued weight loss (or maintenance) regime, when you'll 'fall off the wagon'. This is entirely normal – we're all human. You might overindulge during a festive season or while on holiday. Stressful times can also trigger many people to overeat (which again is completely normal and human), and as a result gain some weight. When these situations arise, I suggest you switch back to the attack phase, even if it's just for a few days or a week – however long you need until you lose the weight you gained, and get yourself back on track. That's how I designed The Food Effect diet – the two phases allow enough flexibility to acknowledge and accommodate real life.

For ease, while all the options that follow are for The Food Effect lifestyle phase, I've also given some that are suitable for the attack phase, so that if you wish to choose 'stricter' options for certain meals (for example, if you've got a big dinner in the evening and want to be more 'careful' for breakfast and lunch), you can simply choose an option that is 'attack-phase friendly'. That way you'll stay on track easily, throughout your new way of life.

BREAKFAST

Attack-phase recipes for 'stricter' meals

• Perfect Porridge (see recipe page 192)
Served with 75g blueberries/mixed berries, or 1 mini-box (14g) raisins or 1 tbsp mixed seeds (such as sunflower seeds, pumpkin seeds and linseeds)
Coffee or tea with skimmed milk, or herbal tea

• 170g 0% Greek yoghurt – add stevia (optional)
75g mixed berries (blueberries, blackberries, strawberries)
Drizzle of agave syrup (1 tsp)
Coffee or tea with skimmed milk, or herbal tea

• 150g low-fat natural yoghurt – add stevia (optional)
Served with 75g mixed berries, plus 1 tbsp pumpkin/sunflower seeds
Drizzle of agave syrup (1 tsp), plus cinnamon
Coffee or tea with skimmed milk, or herbal tea

• 1 boiled or poached egg
1 slice wholemeal bread, toasted
1 apple or orange, or ½ grapefruit – top with stevia or xylitol
Coffee or tea with skimmed milk, or herbal tea

• 1 boiled or poached egg
1 slice wholemeal toast or 3 Ryvita
Sliced fresh tomato or 2 grilled tomato halves, seasoned with salt
and pepper
Coffee or tea with skimmed milk, or herbal tea

• Eggs with Greens:
Scramble or poach 2 eggs and serve with unlimited spinach/rocket/
steamed green beans
Coffee or tea with skimmed milk, or herbal tea

• Smoked Salmon Omelette (see recipe page 194)
Served with fresh sliced tomatoes (unlimited) or 150g sliced
strawberries
Coffee or tea with skimmed milk, or herbal tea

• 1 slice wholemeal toast or 3 Ryvita
120g low-fat cottage cheese
150g strawberries/mixed berries
Coffee or tea with skimmed milk, or herbal tea

• 1 slice wholemeal toast or 3 Ryvita
120g low-fat cottage cheese
Sliced fresh tomato, seasoned with herbs, salt and pepper
Coffee or tea with skimmed milk, or herbal tea

• Smoked Salmon on Toast:
1 slice wholemeal or rye bread, toasted
60g smoked salmon
Sliced cucumber or tomato, with lemon juice, salt and pepper
1 apple or pear
Coffee or tea with skimmed milk, or herbal tea

• Quick and Easy Vegetable Omelette or Scramble (see recipe page 195)
3 Ryvita crackers or 1 slice wholemeal toast
Coffee or tea with skimmed milk, or herbal tea

• Coconut French Toast (see recipe page 194)
Served with 75g strawberries, sliced
Coffee or tea with skimmed milk, or herbal tea

• Avocado Toast (see recipe page 193)
Served with fresh sliced tomato
Coffee or tea with skimmed milk, or herbal tea

Lifestyle-phase recipes

• Porridge cooked in microwave using 1 packet instant oats (no added sugar), or ½ cup uncooked oats, plus 180ml skimmed or almond milk, stevia and a pinch of salt (allow to stand for a few minutes before eating – it swells)
Once cooked add 1 tbsp peanut or almond butter, stevia and cinnamon
Coffee or tea with skimmed milk, or herbal tea

• 2 Weetabix/Oatibix, topped with stevia and cinnamon
240ml skimmed or almond milk
1 mini (14g) box (2 tbsp) raisins
Coffee or tea with skimmed milk, or herbal tea

• 40g whole-grain cereal (such as All-Bran or Bran Flakes)
240ml skimmed or almond milk
Blueberries
Coffee or tea with skimmed milk, or herbal tea

• 125g low-fat or fat-free natural yoghurt – add stevia and cinnamon
25g All-Bran or Bran Flakes
75g blueberries or 2 tbsp (1 mini box, or 14g) raisins
Coffee or tea with skimmed milk, or herbal tea

• Almond Mango Yoghurt:
150g low-fat natural or soya yoghurt
Topped with 75g chopped fresh mango and 1 tbsp toasted flaked almonds
Drizzle of agave syrup (1–2 tsp), plus sprinkling of ginger/cinnamon
Coffee or tea with skimmed milk, or herbal tea

• 125g low-fat natural yoghurt – add stevia or xylitol
150g fruit (such as cut-up melon, pineapple, strawberries or other berries)
3 Ryvita crackers or 1 slice wholemeal toast
Coffee or tea with skimmed milk, or herbal tea

• 1 slice wholemeal toast or 3 Ryvita crackers
120g low-fat cottage cheese mixed with stevia and cinnamon
150g diced pineapple (or any fruit, such as strawberries and melon)
Coffee or tea with skimmed milk, or herbal tea

• ½ wholemeal bagel or 1 slice wholemeal toast
1 tbsp low-fat cream cheese, plus 2 slices smoked salmon (with lemon juice, salt and pepper)

Sliced cucumber
Coffee or tea with skimmed milk, or herbal tea

• ½ wholemeal bagel or 1 slice wholemeal toast
1 tbsp peanut butter
1 apple
Coffee or tea with skimmed milk, or herbal tea

• Nutty Vanilla Overnight Oats (see recipe page 196)
Coffee or tea with skimmed milk, or herbal tea

• Protein Parfait (see recipe page 196)
Coffee or tea with skimmed milk, or herbal tea

• Two-ingredient Sweet Potato Protein Pancakes (see recipe page 197)
Served with 2 tbsp natural yoghurt, stevia, cinnamon and blueberries
Coffee or tea with skimmed milk, or herbal tea

• 1 Home-made Wholesome Energy Bar (see recipe page 198)
1 large apple
Coffee or tea with skimmed milk, or herbal tea

• 1 Guilt-free Courgette Muffin (see recipe page 198)
1 large apple
Coffee or tea with skimmed milk, or herbal tea

• 1 All-natural Skinny Blueberry Muffin (see recipe page 200)
1 large apple
Coffee or tea with skimmed milk, or herbal tea

• Guilt-free Chocolate Protein Pudding (see recipe page 200)
150g blueberries or strawberries
Coffee or tea with skimmed milk, or herbal tea

• The Food Effect Green Power Shake (see recipe page 201)

• The Food Effect Chocolate Green Power Shake (see recipe page 202)

• Sweet Potato Pie Smoothie (see recipe page 203)

MID-MORNING

• Tea, coffee or herbal tea

LUNCH

Attack-phase recipes for 'stricter' meals

• Cottage Cheese Salad:
120g low-fat cottage cheese
Mixed salad/vegetables (lettuce/spinach leaves, tomatoes, cucumber, grated carrot, red/yellow pepper), seasoned with balsamic vinegar or lemon juice, salt and pepper
3 Ryvita crackers or brown rice cakes, or 1 slice wholemeal toast

• Smoked Salmon and Avocado Salad:
2 slices smoked salmon (60g), plus ½ avocado (cubed/sliced)
Mixed salad (lettuce/spinach leaves, cherry tomatoes, cucumber, grated carrot, red/yellow pepper), tossed with balsamic vinegar or lemon juice, salt and pepper
3 Ryvita crackers or brown rice cakes, or 1 slice wholemeal or rye toast

• Tuna Salad:
½ regular size tin of tuna (60g) (in water or brine), mixed with 1 tbsp low-fat mayonnaise
Mixed salad/vegetables (lettuce/spinach leaves, cherry tomatoes, cucumber, grated carrot, red/yellow pepper, red onion), tossed with balsamic vinegar or lemon juice, salt and pepper
3 Ryvita crackers or brown rice cakes, or 1 slice wholemeal toast

• Tuna and Sweetcorn Salad:
½ regular size tin of tuna (60g) (in water or brine), mixed with 1 tbsp low-fat mayonnaise
1 small tin of sweetcorn (150g)
Mixed salad/vegetables (lettuce/spinach leaves, cucumber, cherry tomatoes, grated carrot, red/yellow pepper), tossed with balsamic vinegar or lemon juice, and salt and pepper

• Mackerel Salad:
1 tin of mackerel in tomato sauce (125g)
Mixed salad/spinach leaves
½ red pepper, sliced, chopped cucumber, plus 1 chopped tomato
Season with lemon juice, salt and pepper

• Mixed Bean Salad:
Combine 1 small tin (150g) or ½ regular tin of mixed bean salad, 1 red pepper, diced or 2 chopped tomatoes and unlimited mixed salad leaves
Drizzle with balsamic vinegar, plus herbs, salt and black pepper
On the side: 1 large apple or pear, or serve with 3 Ryvita or brown rice cakes

• Quinoa, Feta and Avocado Salad:
185g cooked quinoa
60g reduced-fat feta cheese
Diced cucumber, tomato, red pepper and ¼ avocado
Top with lemon juice, salt and pepper

• Quinoa Tuna Salad:
185g cooked quinoa
½ tin of tuna (60g) (in water or brine)
Mixed salad (diced cucumber, tomato and red pepper)
1 tbsp low-fat mayo, and lemon juice, salt and pepper

• Smoked Salmon Sandwich on Rye:
Spread 2 slices rye bread with mustard and add:
2 slices smoked salmon, plus a handful of fresh spinach leaves, and lemon juice, salt and pepper
Pre-cut carrot sticks – on the side (unlimited)

• Chicken/Salmon Salad:
Combine 150g cooked (grilled) chicken breast or salmon fillet, unlimited mixed salad greens, 10 cherry tomatoes, plus 1 sliced spring onion
Top with balsamic vinegar, plus herbs, salt and black pepper
On the side: 1 apple or pear

• Quinoa Salad with Roasted Vegetables (see recipe page 203) – use leftovers from dinner
1 large apple

• Roasted Vegetable and Chickpea Salad (see recipe page 205)

• Spicy Tomato and Pepper Frittata (see recipe page 205) – use leftovers from dinner
Serve with mixed green salad, plus balsamic vinegar

• Avocado, Spinach and Strawberry Salad with Sweet Poppy Seed Dressing (see recipe page 208)

• The Food Effect Skinny Chicken Salad Deluxe (see recipe page 210)

• Mediterranean Salad (see recipe page 204)

• Avocado and Cottage Cheese Salad (see recipe page 207)

• The Food Effect Greek Salad (see recipe page 209)

Lifestyle-phase recipes

• Smoked Salmon, Cucumber and Cream Cheese Sandwich:
Sandwich/open toast made with 2 slices wholemeal or rye bread
2 slices smoked salmon (60g), plus 2 tbsp low-fat cream cheese and
sliced cucumber
Lemon juice, salt and pepper
Pre-cut carrot sticks – on the side (unlimited)

• Smoked Salmon, Tomato and Avocado Sandwich:
Sandwich made with 2 slices wholemeal or rye bread
2 slices smoked salmon (60g)
¼ avocado and fresh tomato, sliced
Lemon juice, salt and pepper
Pre-cut carrot sticks – on the side (unlimited)

• Tuna Salad Sandwich:
Sandwich made with 2 pieces wholemeal bread
½ tin of tuna (60g), plus 1 tbsp low-fat mayonnaise
Spinach leaves and sliced tomato, plus salt and pepper
Pre-cut carrot sticks – on the side

• 1 whole-wheat pitta or 2 slices wholemeal bread
Filled with salad (fresh spinach leaves) and sliced tomato, seasoned
with herbs, salt and pepper
2 tbsp reduced-fat hummus
Pre-cut carrot sticks – on the side

• Whole-wheat pitta or 2 slices wholemeal bread
Filled with salad (fresh spinach leaves), plus sliced cucumber/
tomato
1 boiled egg, sliced/mashed, plus 1 tbsp low-fat mayonnaise
Pre-cut carrot sticks – on the side

• 125g cooked couscous (whole wheat)
60g reduced-fat feta cheese
Mixed salad (diced cucumber, tomato, red pepper and so on)
Dressed with 1 tbsp tahini mixed with 1–2 tbsp lemon juice, plus salt
and black pepper

• 4 Corn Thins
110g low-fat cottage cheese
Topped with sliced cucumber or tomato
1 apple or pear

• 2 Ryvita
110g low-fat cottage cheese
Mixed salad (diced cucumber, tomato and so on)
¼ avocado

• 4 Ryvita or brown rice cakes, topped with:
2 boiled eggs (discard 1 yolk), sliced or mashed, plus 1 tbsp low-fat
mayonnaise
Sliced fresh tomato, seasoned with salt and black pepper
Pre-cut carrot sticks – on the side (unlimited)

• Wild Rice and Avocado Salad:
Combine unlimited salad leaves, a large chunk of chopped
cucumber, 1–2 spring onions, 1 grated or chopped raw carrot,
½ sliced avocado, fresh coriander and 125g cooked wild or
brown rice. Season with salt and pepper. Dress with lemon juice or
balsamic vinegar.

• Avocado and Almond Salad (see recipe page 213)

• Eggs in a Mug (see recipe page 222)
3 Ryvita crackers or 1 slice wholemeal toast

• Spinach Salad with Strawberries (see recipe page 212)

• 1 serving Protein-packed Pasta Dish (see recipe page 217)

• 1 serving Curried Chicken Salad (see recipe page 219)
Fresh salad greens (unlimited), plus 3 Ryvita

• Tuscan-style Tuna Bean Salad (see recipe page 223)

• Quinoa Salad with Avocado, Mango and Pomegranate (see recipe page 231)

SOUPS AND SIDES

• 1 large bowl of soup (see recipes – choose one from Lentil/Pea/Carrot, Ginger and Sweet Potato/Tomato/Gorgeously Green Soup) served with one small wholemeal roll and a green side salad

MID-AFTERNOON SNACKS

Attack-phase recipes for 'stricter' snacks

• 1 apple or pear, plus 2 Ryvita crackers, brown rice cakes or oatcakes
Mug of coffee or tea with skimmed milk, or herbal tea

• 1 apple, plus 1 tbsp (15g) peanut or almond butter
Mug of coffee or tea with skimmed milk, or herbal tea

• 2 sticks of celery topped with 2 tbsp low-fat cottage cheese
Mug of coffee or tea with skimmed milk, or herbal tea

• 1 apple or pear, plus 1 handful (12) almonds or 30 pistachio nuts
Mug of coffee or tea with skimmed milk, or herbal tea

• 1 orange, plus 1 handful (12) almonds or cashew nuts
Mug of coffee or tea with skimmed milk, or herbal tea

• 1 apple or pear, plus 1 handful (12) almonds or cashew nuts
Mug of coffee or tea with skimmed milk, or herbal tea

• 150g strawberries, plus 12 almonds
Mug of coffee or tea with skimmed milk, or herbal tea

• 2 dried figs, plus 1 handful (12) almonds or 1 tbsp pumpkin seeds
Mug of coffee or tea with skimmed milk, or herbal tea

• Pre-cut carrot sticks, plus 2 tbsp (30g) reduced-fat hummus
Mug of coffee or tea with skimmed milk, or herbal tea

• 2 Ryvita crackers, brown rice cakes or oatcakes, plus 2 tbsp (30g)
reduced-fat hummus
Mug of coffee or tea with skimmed milk, or herbal tea

• 2 Ryvita crackers or brown rice cakes, plus 2 tbsp low-fat cream
cheese or cottage cheese
Mug of coffee or tea with skimmed milk, or herbal tea

• 2 brown rice cakes or oatcakes, plus 1 tbsp (15g) peanut butter
Mug of coffee or tea with skimmed milk, or herbal tea

• 150g low-fat natural yoghurt, plus 75g fresh blueberries, with
stevia and cinnamon
Mug of coffee or tea with skimmed milk, or herbal tea

• 150g low-fat natural yoghurt, plus 75g strawberries, with stevia
and cinnamon
Mug of coffee or tea with skimmed milk, or herbal tea

Lifestyle-phase snacks

• 1 large apple, plus 1 boiled egg
Mug of coffee or tea with skimmed milk, or herbal tea

• 2 tbsp mixed nuts and 1 plum
Mug of coffee or tea with skimmed milk, or herbal tea

• Small bunch red grapes (50g), plus 12 almonds or 30 pistachio nuts
Mug of coffee or tea with skimmed milk, or herbal tea

• 1 mini-box (14g) raisins, plus 1 handful (12) unsalted almonds or cashew nuts
Mug of coffee or tea with skimmed milk, or herbal tea

• 2 tangerines or plums, plus 1 handful (12) unsalted almonds or cashew nuts
Mug of coffee or tea with skimmed milk, or herbal tea

• 5 dried apricots or prunes, plus 1 handful (12) almonds
Mug of coffee or tea with skimmed milk, or herbal tea

• 3 prunes or dried apricots, plus 6 walnuts
Mug of coffee or tea with skimmed milk, or herbal tea

• 2 tangerines, plus 1 tbsp pumpkin seeds
Mug of coffee or tea with skimmed milk, or herbal tea

• 1 Nākd bar (35g size), plus 1 apple
Mug of coffee or tea with skimmed milk, or herbal tea

• Carrot, celery, cucumber and red pepper crudités, plus 2 tbsp reduced-fat hummus
Mug of coffee or tea with skimmed milk, or herbal tea

• 2 brown rice cakes, Ryvita crackers or Corn Thins, plus ½ avocado
Mug of coffee or tea with skimmed milk, or herbal tea

• 2 oatcakes each topped with 1 tbsp guacamole
Mug of coffee or tea with skimmed milk, or herbal tea

• 150g low-fat natural yoghurt, plus 1 apple or 2 plums
Mug of coffee or tea with skimmed milk, or herbal tea

• 150g low-fat natural yoghurt, plus 1 nectarine or a small bunch of grapes
Mug of coffee or tea with skimmed milk, or herbal tea

• 30g low-fat (salted) popcorn
Mug of coffee or tea with skimmed milk, or herbal tea

• 1 medium skinny latte
1 large apple or pear

• 1 Guilt-free Courgette Muffin (see recipe page 198)
Mug of coffee or tea with skimmed milk, or herbal tea

• 1 All-natural Skinny Blueberry Muffin (see recipe page 200)
Mug of coffee or tea with skimmed milk, or herbal tea

• 1–2 All-healthy Raw Chocolate Truffle Balls (see recipe page 237), plus 1 apple
Mug of coffee or tea with skimmed milk, or herbal tea

• 1–2 Raw Bakewell Tart Balls (see recipe page 238), plus 1 apple
Mug of coffee or tea with skimmed milk, or herbal tea

• 1 Sweet and Healthy Hummus Muffin (see recipe page 238)
Mug of coffee or tea with skimmed milk, or herbal tea

• 1 Fudgy Flourless Peanut Butter Hummus Bar (see recipe page 240), plus 1 apple
Mug of coffee or tea with skimmed milk, or herbal tea

• 1 No-bake Fibre-filled Brownie Bar (see recipe page 240), plus 1 apple
Mug of coffee or tea with skimmed milk, or herbal tea

• 1–2 Raw Peanut Cookie Energy Balls (see recipe page 241), plus 1 apple
Mug of coffee or tea with skimmed milk, or herbal tea

• 1–2 Tropical Mango Energy Balls (see recipe page 242), plus 1 apple or 150g pineapple or mango
Mug of coffee or tea with skimmed milk, or herbal tea

DINNERS

Attack-phase recipes for 'stricter' meals

• 1 grilled or baked chicken breast (150g) or roasted chicken thigh (no skin)
Fresh spinach/salad greens, drizzled with balsamic vinegar
Diced fresh tomatoes/red pepper, seasoned with salt and pepper
125g cooked quinoa or whole-wheat couscous

• Honey-roasted Chicken:
Top 1 chicken breast with 1 tbsp honey and soya sauce, and grill
Serve with unlimited steamed broccoli and/or cauliflower

• Easy Roast Supper:
Rotisserie chicken breast (150g)
Roasted vegetables such as courgettes, mushrooms, red peppers and red onions, cooked with minimal oil or spray oil, and seasoned with herbs, garlic powder, salt and pepper
1 small baked sweet potato (150g) or Miraculous Butternut Squash Mash (see recipe page 225)

• Teriyaki Salmon:
Marinate 1 fillet of salmon (180g) in 3 tbsp soya sauce, 1 tsp
olive oil, 1 tsp finely grated ginger and 1 tsp honey or agave
syrup. Preheat oven to 200°C/Gas 6. Place the salmon, coated
in marinade, on a baking tray lined with foil and bake in oven for
10–12 minutes until cooked through.
Serve with unlimited mixed stir-fried or roasted vegetables (in minimal
oil/spray oil)

• Turkey-stuffed Peppers (see recipe page 212)

• Baked Sweet Potato with Beetroot and Cottage Cheese (see recipe
page 209)

• Smoked Salmon Omelette (see recipe page 194)
Served with fresh salad greens (unlimited)

• Quick and Easy Vegetable Omelette or Scramble (see recipe)
Served with 1 slice wholemeal toast or 3 Ryvita Dark Rye crackers
Fresh salad greens (unlimited)

• Spicy Tomato and Pepper Frittata (see recipe page 205) – save
half for lunch
Served with large mixed green salad drizzled with balsamic vinegar

• Chinese Chicken Stir-fry (see recipe page 211)
Served with 125g cooked brown rice
Mixed green salad drizzled with balsamic vinegar

• Spicy Stuffed Sweet Potato (see recipe page 206)
Served with fresh spinach leaves/mixed green salad drizzled with
balsamic vinegar

• Avocado and Cottage Cheese Salad (see recipe page 207)

• Quinoa Salad with Roasted Vegetables (see recipe page 203)
Served with mixed green salad drizzled with balsamic vinegar

• The Food Effect Skinny Chicken Salad Deluxe (see recipe page 210)

• Chicken, Spinach and Strawberry Salad with Sweet Poppy Seed
Dressing (see recipe page 207)

• Avocado, Spinach and Strawberry Salad with Sweet Poppy Seed
Dressing (see recipe page 208)
Served with 60g smoked salmon

Lifestyle-phase recipes

• 1 grilled or baked chicken breast (150g) or roasted chicken thigh
(no skin)
Steamed or roasted green beans/broccoli/cauliflower/asparagus,
seasoned with garlic powder, herbs, salt and pepper (unlimited), or
Miraculous Cauliflower Mash (see recipe page 224)
125g (cooked) brown rice or ½ baked sweet potato

• Cajun Chicken Breast with Red Cabbage Slaw (see recipe page 214)
Served with 125g (cooked) brown rice or quinoa

• Cajun Chicken Breast Pitta (see recipe page 215)
Served with mixed green salad and balsamic vinegar on the side

• 1 grilled chicken breast (150g) or roasted chicken thigh (no skin)
Roasted vegetables such as green beans, mushrooms, red onions
and courgette, with minimal oil or spray oil, seasoned with herbs,
garlic powder, salt and pepper
Fresh spinach leaves drizzled with low-sodium soya sauce or
balsamic vinegar
125g cooked couscous (whole-wheat) or quinoa

• 1 vegetarian burger
Roasted vegetables such as courgettes, mushrooms, red peppers and
red onions, cooked with minimal oil or spray oil, and seasoned with
herbs, garlic powder, salt and pepper
1 small baked sweet potato (150g) or Miraculous Butternut Squash
Mash (see recipe page 225)

• 1 grilled or baked salmon fillet (150g), seasoned with lemon juice,
soya sauce and herbs
Steamed or roasted green beans, broccoli, cauliflower or asparagus
(unlimited), seasoned with garlic powder, herbs, salt and pepper or
Miraculous Cauliflower Mash (see recipe page 224)
125g cooked brown rice or ½ baked sweet potato

• 1 grilled or baked salmon fillet (150g), seasoned with lemon juice,
soya sauce and herbs
Fresh spinach/salad greens, drizzled with low-sodium soya sauce or
balsamic vinegar
Diced fresh tomatoes, with herbs, salt and pepper
125g cooked couscous (whole wheat), or quinoa or brown rice

• 1 grilled or baked salmon fillet (150g), seasoned with lemon juice,
soya sauce and herbs
Served with 1 serving Winning Combo Salad (see recipe page 230)

• 1 grilled or baked chicken breast (150g) or cooked/roasted
chicken (no skin)
Served with 1 serving Winning Combo Salad (see recipe page 230)

• 1 vegetarian burger
Served with 1 serving Winning Combo Salad (see recipe page 230)

• Tuna Steak with Quinoa and Spinach:
1 grilled tuna steak (150g)
150g cooked quinoa

Fresh baby spinach leaves, drizzled with lemon juice, soya sauce or balsamic vinegar

• 1 tuna steak (150g)
Mixed salad (baby spinach leaves, cherry tomatoes, cucumber, grated carrot, beetroot and chopped red or yellow pepper)
125g cooked brown rice

• 1 vegetarian burger
1 whole-wheat pitta
Lettuce and sliced tomato
Mustard and ketchup
Served with mixed green salad and balsamic vinegar on the side

• 1 vegetarian burger
Steamed or roasted green beans, broccoli, cauliflower or asparagus (unlimited), seasoned with garlic powder, herbs, salt and pepper or Miraculous Cauliflower Mash (see recipe page 224)
125g cooked brown rice or ½ baked sweet potato

• 1 vegetarian burger
Fresh spinach/salad greens, drizzled with balsamic vinegar
Diced fresh tomatoes/red pepper, seasoned with salt and pepper
125g cooked couscous (whole wheat) or quinoa

• 1 lean steak (150g)
Steamed green beans/broccoli or fresh salad/spinach leaves, unlimited
½ baked sweet potato, or 125g cooked brown rice or corn on the cob, or Miraculous Butternut Squash Mash (see recipe page 225)
Ketchup, to serve

• 1 medium-sized baked sweet potato (200g)
1 small tin of baked beans or 110g low-fat cottage cheese
Mixed green salad, plus diced tomato wedges, seasoned with salt and pepper, and drizzled with balsamic vinegar

• 1 medium-sized baked sweet potato (200g)
½ tin of tuna (60g) (in water or brine), plus 1 tbsp low-fat
mayonnaise
Mixed green salad, plus diced tomato wedges, seasoned with salt
and pepper, and drizzled with balsamic vinegar

• Whole-wheat pasta (70g uncooked)
120g low-fat cottage cheese, or ½ tin of tuna (in water or brine), or
½ chicken breast (100g), sliced
240ml ready-made tomato pasta sauce ('Marinara')
Served on top of a large bowl of fresh spinach leaves or steamed
green beans

• 1 large bowl Healthy Hearty Minestrone – a 'meal in a bowl' (see
recipe page 215)
Pre-cut carrot or other vegetable sticks on the side (unlimited)

• 1 large bowl of soup (see recipes – choose one from Red Lentil/Pea/
Carrot, Ginger and Sweet Potato/Tomato/Gorgeously Green Soup)
Served with 1 small wholemeal roll and green side salad

• Hummus Chicken (see recipe page 216)
Served with 125g cooked brown rice, plus chopped cucumber and
tomato salad or mixed green salad (unlimited)

• 1 serving Protein-packed Pasta Dish (see recipe page 217)

• 1 serving Vegetable Bolognaise (see recipe page 218)

• Saucy Salmon and Veggie Bake (see recipe page 222)

• 2–3 Salmon and Sweet Potato Sliders with Roasted Red Pepper
Sauce (see recipe page 220)
Served with unlimited fresh salad/spinach leaves and sliced tomato
seasoned with herbs, salt and pepper

• Tuscan-style Tuna Bean Salad (see recipe page 223)

• 1 grilled or baked chicken breast or 150g fillet of salmon (or any fish)
Fresh spinach/salad greens, drizzled with balsamic vinegar
1 serving Quinoa Salad with Avocado, Mango and Pomegranate (see recipe page 231)

• 1 vegetarian burger
Fresh spinach/salad greens, drizzled with balsamic vinegar
1 serving Quinoa Salad with Avocado, Mango and Pomegranate (see recipe page 231)

• 1 grilled or baked chicken breast or 150g fillet of salmon (or any fish)
Fresh spinach/salad greens, drizzled with balsamic vinegar
1 serving Rainbow Brown Rice Salad (see recipe page 232)

• 1 vegetarian burger
Fresh spinach/salad greens, drizzled with balsamic vinegar
1 serving Rainbow Brown Rice Salad (see recipe page 232)

• 1 grilled or baked chicken breast or 150g fillet of salmon (or any fish)
Fresh spinach/salad greens, drizzled with balsamic vinegar
1 serving Quinoa Tabbouleh Salad (see recipe page 233)

• 1 vegetarian burger
Fresh spinach/salad greens, drizzled with balsamic vinegar
1 serving Quinoa Tabbouleh Salad (see recipe page 233)

AFTER DINNER OR LATE-EVENING SNACKS

Drink herbal tea, and opt for any of the following snack options.

Attack-phase recipes for 'stricter' snacks

• 30g dark chocolate (70 per cent cocoa or above), plus fruit such as 1 apple or pear, or 150g strawberries or 1 orange

• Baked Apple with Pecan Nuts:
1 baked (or fresh if preferred) apple, sprinkled with stevia, cinnamon and 2 tbsp chopped pecan nuts

• Strawberries with Pecan Nuts:
75g sliced strawberries, plus 1 tbsp crushed pecan nuts

• Pear with Pecan Nuts:
Serve ½ a baked pear (or fresh if preferred), sprinkled with stevia and cinnamon, plus 1 tbsp crushed pecan nuts

• Fresh fruit (apple, pear or orange), plus 15 almonds

• 25g mixed dried fruit and nuts

• 1 low-fat natural yoghurt (150g), plus 150g strawberries or blueberries, and stevia and cinnamon

• 2 oatcakes or Ryvita crackers, plus 2 tbsp reduced-fat hummus

Lifestyle-phase snacks

• Apple with Almond Butter:
Slice 1 apple thinly and spread slices with almond butter (1 tbsp total)

• Apple with Peanut Butter:
Slice 1 apple thinly or into wedges, and spread slices with peanut butter (1 tbsp total)

• 1 Nākd bar (35g size), plus 1 serving fresh fruit

• 1 low-fat natural yoghurt (150g), plus 1 nectarine or bunch of grapes

• 2 Flourless Peanut Butter Biscuits (see recipe page 236), plus 1 fruit (such as apple or orange)

• 1–2 All-healthy Raw Chocolate Truffle Balls (see recipe page 237), plus 1 serving fruit (such as 1 apple or orange, 150g melon or strawberries, or small bunch of grapes)

• 1–2 Raw Bakewell Tart Balls (see recipe page 238), plus 1 serving fruit (such as 1 apple or orange, 150g melon or strawberries)

• Guilt-free Chocolate Protein Pudding (see recipe page 200), plus 75g fresh blueberries or strawberries

• 1 Chocolate Peanut Cluster (see recipe page 239), plus 1 serving fruit (such as 1 apple or orange, 150g melon or strawberries, or small bunch of grapes)

• 1 Fudgy Flourless Peanut Butter Hummus Bar (see recipe page 240), plus 1 serving fruit (such as 1 apple or orange, 150g melon or strawberries, or small bunch of grapes)

• 1 No-bake Fibre-filled Brownie Bar (see recipe page 240), plus 1 serving fruit (such as 1 apple or orange, 150g melon or strawberries, or small bunch of grapes)

• 1–2 Raw Peanut Cookie Energy Balls (see recipe page 241),
plus 1 serving fruit (such as 1 apple or orange, 150g melon or
strawberries, or small bunch of grapes)

• 1–2 Tropical Mango Energy Balls (see recipe page 242),
plus 1 serving fruit (such as 1 apple or orange, 150g melon or
strawberries, or small bunch of grapes)

• 1 slice Flourless Carrot Cake (see recipe page 242), plus 1 serving
fresh fruit

CHAPTER 13

The Food Effect Recipes

Simple, healthy, delicious

In this chapter you'll find all the recipes specified in both the attack and lifestyle phases of The Food Effect meal plan and the options given in Chapters 11 and 12. All the recipes are super-simple, quick and easy to prepare, demonstrating that preparing healthy food doesn't require you to spend hours cooking in the kitchen.

For practical purposes, most of the recipes serve one or two people – those that make two portions are often included in the next day's lunch or dinner, so that leftovers can be put to good use. Recipes can of course also be doubled if you're doing the plan along with a friend or partner, or if you are feeding family or friends.

The recipes are listed below for your convenience so that you can 'pick and choose' to fit in with the plan. **All the options are suitable for The Food Effect lifestyle phase, while only those with an asterisk can be eaten during the attack phase.** When you have adopted this as your new way of eating, you can of course still choose options from the attack phase; for instance, if you're going out for a big dinner and want to be more 'careful' at breakfast and lunch that day. That way you'll stay on track easily.

* indicates an attack-phase recipe

BREAKFASTS

* Perfect Porridge
* Avocado Toast
* Smoked Salmon Omelette
* Coconut French Toast
* Quick and Easy Vegetable Omelette or Scramble
Nutty Vanilla Overnight Oats
Protein Parfait
Two-ingredient Sweet Potato Protein Pancakes
Home-made Wholesome Energy Bars
Guilt-free Courgette Muffins
All-natural Skinny Blueberry Muffins
Guilt-free Chocolate Protein Pudding
The Food Effect Green Power Shake
The Food Effect Chocolate Green Power Shake
Sweet Potato Pie Smoothie

LUNCHES AND DINNERS

* Quinoa Salad with Roasted Vegetables
* Mediterranean Salad
* Spicy Tomato and Pepper Frittata
* Roasted Vegetable and Chickpea Salad
* Smoked Salmon Omelette (see 'Breakfasts' for recipe)
* Spicy Stuffed Sweet Potato
* Avocado and Cottage Cheese Salad
* Quick and Easy Vegetable Omelette or Scramble (see 'Breakfasts' for recipe)
* Chicken, Spinach and Strawberry Salad with Sweet Poppy Seed Dressing
* Avocado, Spinach and Strawberry Salad with Sweet Poppy Seed Dressing
* Baked Sweet Potato with Beetroot and Cottage Cheese
* The Food Effect Greek Salad

* The Food Effect Skinny Chicken Salad Deluxe
* Chinese Chicken Stir-fry
* Turkey Stuffed Peppers
Spinach Salad with Strawberries
Avocado and Almond Salad
Quinoa Salad with Avocado, Mango and Pomegranate (See 'Side Dishes' for recipe)
Cajun Chicken Breast with Red Cabbage Slaw
Cajun Chicken Breast Pitta
Healthy Hearty Minestrone
Hummus Chicken
Protein-packed Pasta Dish
Vegetable Bolognaise
Curried Chicken Salad
Salmon and Sweet Potato Sliders with Roasted Red Pepper Sauce
Eggs in a Mug
Saucy Salmon and Veggie Bake
Tuscan-style Tuna Bean Salad

SOUPS AND SIDE DISHES

* Miraculous Cauliflower Mash
* Miraculous Butternut Squash Mash
The Food Effect World Cup Pea Soup
Easiest Ever Red Lentil Soup
Carrot, Ginger and Sweet Potato Soup
Gorgeously Green Soup
Fresh Tomato Soup with Mixed Green Pesto
Healthy Hearty Minestrone (see 'Lunches and Dinners' for recipe)
Winning Combo Salad
Red Cabbage Slaw
Quinoa Salad with Avocado, Mango and Pomegranate
Rainbow Brown Rice Salad
Quinoa Tabbouleh Salad

SNACKS AND SWEET TREATS

* Healthy Home-made Peanut Butter
* Best-ever Healthy Home-made Hummus
Guilt-free Courgette Muffins (see 'Breakfasts' for recipe)
Flourless Peanut Butter Biscuits
All-healthy Raw Chocolate Truffle Balls
Guilt-free Chocolate Protein Pudding (see 'Breakfasts' for recipe)
Raw Bakewell Tart Balls
Sweet and Healthy Hummus Muffins
Chocolate Peanut Clusters
Fudgy Flourless Peanut Butter Hummus Bars
No-bake Fibre-filled Brownie Bars
Raw Peanut Cookie Energy Balls
Tropical Mango Energy Balls
Flourless Carrot Cake

Note: During the twenty-eight day attack phase, follow the specific serving/topping suggestions in the plan. Once you reach your goal weight (during the lifestyle phase), you can be more flexible and creative.

BREAKFASTS

Perfect Porridge

This is delicious topped with 1 tablespoon of the following: sunflower seeds/pumpkin seeds/flaked almonds/peanut butter/almond butter, plus fresh blueberries, strawberries or mixed berries.

Serves 1

40g rolled oats
180ml skimmed, soya or almond milk

2 tsp stevia or xylitol
Pinch of salt
½ tsp cinnamon

Place the oats and cooking liquid in a small pot. Cook over a medium heat, uncovered, for around 5 minutes – stirring as the oats thicken and reach the desired consistency (add more water if necessary). Once the oats are cooked and creamy, add the stevia, salt and cinnamon. Stir and remove from the heat. Spoon the porridge into a bowl. Allow to stand for a few minutes before eating – it swells and gets much better.

Avocado Toast

A classic favourite.

Serves 1

1 small or ½ large ripe avocado
1 tbsp lemon juice or juice of ½ lemon
1 tomato
Salt and pepper
Paprika
1 slice wholemeal or rye bread, toasted
Chilli powder/flakes, optional

Slice the avocado in half and remove the stone. Scoop the flesh into a bowl and mash roughly with a fork, adding the lemon juice. Dice the tomato finely. Add to the bowl. Season generously with salt, pepper and paprika. Mix together well.

Top the toast with the avocado mixture. Sprinkle with chilli (if desired).

Smoked Salmon Omelette

Serves 1

1 whole egg
2 egg whites
1 tbsp fresh chopped dill or 1 tsp dried dill
Salt and pepper, to taste
½ tbsp olive oil, for greasing
55g smoked salmon
50g tomato, sliced

Whisk the egg and egg whites with the dill, salt and pepper. Pour the mixture into an oiled, heated frying pan set over a medium flame, to form a thin layer. Allow to cook for about 2 minutes. Lay the smoked salmon and sliced tomato on half the omelette. Fold over the other half of the omelette and serve.

Coconut French Toast

With this recipe, you can eat French Toast for breakfast – or lunch, brunch or dinner! – and stay slim, as it doesn't contain the added sugar, carbs and calories of the standard version. It tastes so decadent and delicious you'll have a hard time believing it's guilt-free and super-good for you, too.

Serves 1

1 egg
1 tbsp skimmed, soya or almond milk
1 slice wholemeal bread (or any bread of your choice, such as spelt or gluten-free)
Desiccated coconut
Coconut oil or cooking spray, for greasing

Granulated stevia or xylitol
Cinnamon
Mixed berries or strawberries, to serve
Agave syrup, to serve

Mix together the egg and milk in a shallow bowl. Dip the bread in the egg mixture to cover fully. Remove the bread from the bowl. Sprinkle the coconut generously over both sides to coat the bread.
Grease a non-stick frying pan lightly with coconut oil or cooking spray, and heat over a medium heat.

Fry the bread on both sides until golden. Transfer to a plate. Sprinkle generously with stevia and cinnamon. Serve with the mixed berries or strawberries alongside, and a drizzle of agave syrup on top.

Quick and Easy Vegetable Omelette or Scramble

Enjoy this with a fresh green salad and some wholemeal toast or crackers.

Serves 1

100g finely sliced vegetables (such as mushrooms, onions, red or yellow pepper or courgettes)
Olive oil cooking spray, or 1 tsp coconut oil
1 whole egg
2 egg whites
1 tsp dried dill (or other herbs)
Salt and pepper, to taste

Lightly sauté the vegetables in the spray oil or coconut oil until soft and set aside. Beat the eggs together with 1 tbsp water, the herbs, salt and pepper. Add to the pan over a low heat and cook gently. When almost set, top with the vegetables. Flip over to heat through. Remove to a plate to serve.

Nutty Vanilla Overnight Oats

Serves 2

100g uncooked porridge oats
240ml skimmed, almond or soya milk (plus additional to serve)
¼ tsp cinnamon
2 tsp stevia or xylitol
½ tsp vanilla essence
Pinch of salt
2 tbsp chopped walnuts (or other nuts of your choice)
Drizzle of agave syrup and fresh berries (such as blueberries), to serve

Combine the oats, milk, cinnamon, stevia, vanilla essence and salt. Stir together, cover and allow to sit in the fridge overnight. In the morning, stir well. Add a splash of extra milk if desired, if you prefer a less thick consistency. Top with the chopped walnuts, fresh berries and a drizzle of agave syrup.

Protein Parfait

Serves 1

200g Greek yoghurt mixed with 1–2 tsp stevia
25g uncooked porridge oats
75g mixed berries (strawberries, blueberries or blackberries)
½ tsp cinnamon
Drizzle of agave syrup (1–2 tsp)

Layer the Greek yoghurt, oats and berries in a large glass or bowl. Sprinkle with the cinnamon and drizzle with agave syrup.

Two-ingredient Sweet Potato Protein Pancakes

These pancakes are all natural, gluten, dairy and sugar free, and provide a filling, nutritious and delicious breakfast. The pancakes can be reheated in the oven.

Makes 6 decent-sized pancakes, serves 2

1 large sweet potato (250g)
6 egg whites, lightly beaten
2 tsp stevia
Cinnamon and salt, to taste
Olive oil cooking spray or 1 tsp coconut oil
Agave syrup, 0% Greek yoghurt and berries, to serve

Cook the sweet potato in the microwave (8 minutes on high) or oven, until completely soft. Scoop out all the flesh into a bowl (discard the skin or eat it separately). Mash the flesh well with a fork. Add the beaten egg whites to the bowl, mixing them in lightly with a fork (any small remaining lumps don't matter). Mix the stevia (or sweetener of your choice), a generous shake of cinnamon and a pinch of salt into the batter.

Use non-stick cooking spray or coconut oil to coat a non-stick frying pan. Heat over a medium heat until hot. Once hot, drop ¼ cup of batter per pancake into the pan. Cook until the edges look firm, around 1 minute. Flip and cook on the other side until fully cooked, around 2 more minutes. Grease the skillet again with oil/spray between cooking batches of pancakes.

To serve, top with your desired toppings, such as agave syrup, natural yoghurt or Greek yoghurt mixed with berries.

Home-made Wholesome Energy Bars

These bars are chewy, filling and delicious. They're packed with protein, fibre and heart-healthy monounsaturated fats and are suitable for vegans, too!

Makes 8 bars

125g uncooked porridge oats (you can use gluten-free oats if required)
140g unsalted almonds
16 Medjool dates, stones removed
20g desiccated coconut (unsweetened)
3 tbsp agave syrup, brown rice syrup or maple syrup
½ tsp almond or vanilla essence
Pinch of salt
120ml water

Preheat the oven to 180°C/Gas 4. Process the oats and almonds in a food processor until finely ground and crumbled. Add the dates, coconut, agave (or alternative) syrup, and almond or vanilla essence and salt, then process again. Add the water slowly, while you process the ingredients together until a thick, sticky, cohesive batter forms.
Spray or grease an 20cm square baking pan and line with baking paper. Spread batter evenly in the pan and press down well with a spatula so that it is firmly packed. Bake in the oven for 20 minutes. Allow to cool. Remove the paper with its contents onto a flat surface, then cut into 8 bars.

Guilt-free Courgette Muffins

These incredibly delicious courgette muffins are full of natural fibre and wholemeal goodness. Courgettes are an excellent 'weight-friendly' food, as they are extremely low in calories, with only 14 per 100g.

The muffins are dairy-free and vegan, so they can be made to suit all dietary requirements. They have a low GI – keeping you fuller for longer and preventing those slumps you get after eating sugary, high-GI white muffins and baked goods.

Makes 8–10 medium-sized muffins

210g whole-wheat (or spelt) flour
½ tsp bicarbonate of soda
¾ tsp salt
1 tsp cinnamon
125g coconut sugar or 62g granulated sweetener, such as stevia
60ml sunflower oil
115g natural apple sauce (no added sugar)
60ml soya milk
1 tsp apple cider or white vinegar
200g grated courgette (1 medium-sized courgette)
45g dark chocolate chips
40g raisins

Preheat the oven to 180°C/Gas 4. Grease a non-stick muffin tray with non-stick cooking oil spray, or line with paper or silicone muffin liners. Combine the dry ingredients (flour, bicarbonate of soda, salt, cinnamon and coconut sugar or sweetener) in one bowl, mix well and set aside.

Combine the oil, apple sauce, soya milk, vinegar and courgette in another bowl. Stir the wet ingredients into the dry ingredients. Add the chocolate chips and raisins. Mix until just combined. Divide the mixture between 8–10 muffin cups. Bake for 20 minutes. Remove from the oven and allow to cool before removing the muffins from the tin.

The muffins can be stored in an airtight container or Ziploc bag for several days at room temperature, or frozen to be enjoyed whenever you fancy.

All-natural Skinny Blueberry Muffins

Bursting with sweet blueberries and packed with natural fibre and whole-grain goodness, these muffins are moist and full of flavour.

Makes 10–12 medium-sized muffins

100g uncooked porridge oats
140g whole-wheat flour
2 tsp bicarbonate of soda
½ tsp cinnamon
¼ tsp salt
125g coconut sugar
1 whole egg
240ml skimmed or soya milk
115g natural apple sauce (no added sugar)
2 tsp vanilla essence
150g blueberries (fresh or frozen*)
* If using frozen blueberries, do not thaw them before adding to the batter.

Preheat the oven to 180°C/Gas 4. Combine the dry ingredients in one bowl, and the remaining ingredients in another. Combine the two and stir together. Mix until just fully combined; do not over-mix. Pour the batter into a greased muffin tray or muffin tray lined with silicone or paper cases, filling each until three-quarters full. Bake for 20–25 minutes, until firm and springy to the touch, or until a toothpick inserted into the muffins comes out clean.

The muffins can be stored in an airtight container or Ziploc bag for several days, or frozen to be enjoyed whenever you fancy.

Guilt-free Chocolate Protein Pudding

This protein-packed pudding is ideal for a mid-afternoon or post-workout snack. It's also delicious eaten as a dip with apple slices or carrot sticks, and even makes the perfect late-night treat when you're craving something sweet.

Serves 1

170g 0% Greek yoghurt
1 tbsp unsweetened cocoa powder
1–2 tbsp agave syrup, to taste (plus extra for drizzling)
¼ tsp vanilla essence
Toppings (optional): blueberries, dark chocolate chips, sliced almonds, dessicated coconut, chopped walnuts

Mix all the ingredients together well in a mixing bowl, until the cocoa powder is fully mixed in, with no lumps left, and a smooth, pudding-like consistency is reached. Spoon into a serving bowl. Top with toppings of your choice. Drizzle with additional agave syrup.
To make the pudding more ice-cream-like, you can pop it in the freezer for 30 minutes before tucking in.

The Food Effect Green Power Shake

Nut-free, dairy-free and vegan options are included in this recipe.

Serves 1

70g frozen chopped spinach
3 handfuls small ice cubes
1–2 scoops (30g) vanilla protein powder*
1 tbsp nut butter (such as peanut or almond butter)**
1 tbsp granulated sweetener (such as stevia)
1 tsp ground cinnamon
¼ tsp ground ginger (optional)
Few drops almond essence (optional, but recommended)
120ml skimmed almond or soya milk

* You can use 30g skimmed milk powder or vegan (soya or pea) protein powder instead

** You can substitute this with ½ avocado for a nut-free version.

Place the frozen spinach and ice in a blender. Blend until the ice is fully crushed (if your blender has an 'ice-crusher' function, use that). Add the remaining ingredients and blend for several minutes on the highest speed until smooth. Pour into a large glass and serve with a straw.

The Food Effect Chocolate Green Power Shake

Dairy-free and vegan options are included in this recipe.

Serves 1

70g frozen chopped spinach
2 handfuls small ice cubes
1–2 scoops (30g) vanilla protein powder*
1 tbsp nut butter (such as peanut or almond butter)
1 tbsp cocoa powder
1–2 tbsp granulated sweetener (such as stevia), to taste
1 tsp ground cinnamon
Few drops mint extract (optional, recommended for chocolate minty version)
120ml skimmed almond or soya milk

*You can substitute this with 30g skimmed milk powder or vegan (soya or pea) protein powder.

Put the spinach and ice in a blender. Blend until the ice is fully crushed (if your blender has an 'ice-crusher' function, use that). Add the rest of the ingredients, and blend for several minutes on the highest speed until smooth. Pour into a large glass and serve with a straw.

Sweet Potato Pie Smoothie

I love shakes and also sweet potatoes, so I've combined the two and come up with this super-simple, sweet and delicious smoothie recipe that's healthy *and* indulgent – it's literally sweet potato pie in a glass!

Serves 1

2 handfuls of ice cubes
1 medium-sized sweet potato, cooked (skin removed)
120ml coconut water
60ml milk of choice (skimmed, soya, almond or coconut)
1 heaped tbsp peanut or almond butter
1–2 tbsp agave syrup, to taste
½ tsp vanilla extract
½ tsp ground cinnamon, plus additional for serving
Pinch of salt

Place the ice in a blender and blend until completely crushed. Add all the remaining ingredients and blend on high speed until smooth. Pour into a tall glass and dust with additional cinnamon. Serve with a straw.

LUNCHES AND DINNERS

Quinoa Salad with Roasted Vegetables

Serves 2

2 small courgettes, chopped
1 medium carrot, chopped
1 small red onion, chopped
380g frozen broccoli or cauliflower
Olive oil, or olive oil cooking spray, for roasting
Salt, pepper and paprika, to taste

130g uncooked quinoa
360ml water, plus generous pinch of salt
Juice of 1 fresh lemon (or 2 tbsp lemon juice)

Lightly coat the vegetables with olive oil. Season well with salt, pepper and paprika. Roast all the vegetables in a preheated oven at 180°C/ Gas 4 until tender, about 20 minutes. Bring the quinoa and salted water to a boil in a medium pot, then reduce the heat to a simmer and cook for 10–15 minutes, or until the water is absorbed and the quinoa is fluffy. Toss everything together in a large serving dish. Serve warm or at room temperature with fresh lemon juice and sea salt to taste.

Mediterranean Salad

For added variety, you can add or interchange ingredients in this recipe. Try blanched green beans, asparagus, ¼ avocado, anchovies, feta cheese, oven-roasted red peppers, aubergines or mushrooms.

Serves 1

2 large handfuls salad greens
1 boiled egg
100g tuna in water or brine (drained weight)
½ cucumber, sliced
1 red onion, sliced
1 large tomato, diced
4 black olives, sliced

Dressing
1 tbsp extra-virgin olive oil
½ tbsp vinegar (balsamic, apple cider or red wine vinegar)
Salt and pepper, to taste

Mix the dressing ingredients in a small bowl, then toss with the salad ingredients.

Spicy Tomato and Pepper Frittata

During the attack phase, this dish is delicious with a fresh green salad and some healthy wholemeal crackers or toast.

Serves 2

Olive oil or spray oil, for cooking
1 red or yellow pepper, diced
2 large vine tomatoes, cubed
1 generous pinch cayenne pepper or dried chilli flakes
½ tsp cumin
Generous pinch of salt and pepper
2 whole eggs
2 egg whites

Lightly grease a frying pan with 1–2 tsp olive oil or cooking oil spray. Heat over a medium heat. Add the pepper, tomatoes, cayenne pepper or chilli flakes, cumin, salt and pepper. Cover the pan with a lid and simmer gently for 5 minutes. Whisk the eggs and egg whites in a bowl and slowly pour them into the pan. Cover and cook over a low heat for 12–15 minutes, or until set. Divide in half and serve.

Roasted Vegetable and Chickpea Salad

Serves 1

280g assorted vegetables for roasting (red onions, courgette, red or yellow pepper, mushrooms and aubergines)
Olive oil or spray oil, for cooking
Herbs, salt and pepper
Mixed salad or spinach leaves
80g tinned chickpeas, drained
50g reduced-fat feta cheese
Balsamic vinegar, mixed herbs, salt and pepper, to serve

Coat your selection of vegetables with spray oil or minimal olive oil, and stir in the herbs, salt and pepper. Put on a baking tray and roast in a preheated 200°C/Gas 6 oven until soft and slightly browned, about 45 minutes. Allow to cool to room temperature or refrigerate for later use.

To prepare the salad, place the mixed salad or spinach leaves on a plate or in a bowl. Add the cooled roasted vegetables. Top with the chickpeas and feta cheese. Drizzle with balsamic vinegar and season with herbs, salt and pepper to taste.

Spicy Stuffed Sweet Potato

Delicious served with a mixed green salad alongside.

Serves 1

1 medium sweet potato (200g)
½ red onion, diced
1 tsp olive oil or cooking spray oil
200g tin kidney beans, drained and rinsed
200g tin chopped tomatoes
1 tbsp tomato purée
½ fresh chilli, deseeded and sliced, or pinch of cayenne pepper or dry chilli flakes
½ tsp paprika
Salt and pepper

Bake the sweet potato in a preheated 190°C/Gas 5 oven until soft (about 1 hour), or in a microwave on high for 7–8 minutes. Fry the onion in a non-stick pan in the olive oil, until softened. Add kidney beans, chopped tomatoes, tomato purée, chilli or chilli powder, paprika, and salt and pepper to taste. Heat through. Serve piled onto the baked sweet potato.

Avocado and Cottage Cheese Salad

Serves 1

Large serving of mixed salad greens—
120g low-fat cottage cheese
Chopped spring onions, to taste
½ avocado
Pinch of chilli powder or cayenne pepper (optional)
Juice of ½ lime or lemon
Salt and pepper, to taste

Place the salad greens on a plate. Scatter with the cottage cheese and spring onions.

Cut the avocado into thin slices or cubes, and scatter over the plate. Sprinkle with a pinch of chilli or cayenne pepper (if using). To serve, dress with lime juice, and season with salt and pepper.

Chicken, Spinach and Strawberry Salad with Sweet Poppy Seed Dressing

See below for a delicious vegetarian option to this recipe.

Serves 1

150g cooked (grilled or baked) chicken breast (no skin)
55g fresh spinach leaves
75g strawberries, hulled and halved
1 tbsp flaked almonds, toasted

Dressing
1 tbsp lemon juice
1 tbsp white vinegar
½ tsp soya sauce

½ tsp olive oil
1 tbsp stevia or xylitol
½ tsp poppy seeds

Chop or slice the chicken breast and set aside. Mix the dressing ingredients and toss through the spinach leaves and strawberries. Fold in the chicken. To serve, arrange on a plate and top with the toasted flaked almonds.

Avocado, Spinach and Strawberry Salad with Sweet Poppy Seed Dressing

This recipe is a variation on the one above. The chicken is replaced with avocado and if you eat fish but not meat you can also serve with 50g smoked salmon.

Serves 1

1 small or ½ large avocado
55g fresh spinach leaves
75g strawberries, hulled and halved
60g smoked salmon (optional)
1 tbsp flaked almonds, toasted

Dressing
1 tbsp lemon juice
1 tbsp white vinegar
½ tsp soya sauce
½ tsp olive oil
1 tbsp stevia or xylitol
½ tsp poppy seeds

Slice or dice the avocado into chunks and set aside. Mix the dressing ingredients and toss through the spinach leaves and strawberries. Fold in the avocado. To serve, arrange the mixture on a plate and top with the smoked salmon (if using) and toasted flaked almonds.

Baked Sweet Potato with Beetroot and Cottage Cheese

Serves 1

1 medium-sized sweet potato (200g)
2–3 whole ready-cooked and peeled beetroot
120g low-fat cottage cheese
Mixed salad greens or spinach leaves
Balsamic vinegar, salt and black pepper

Bake the sweet potato in a preheated 190°C/Gas 5 oven for about 1 hour, or in a microwave on high for 7–8 minutes, until soft. Chop the beetroot into wedges. Sprinkle with salt.

Slice along the potato and split in half. Top with cottage cheese. Season with salt and black pepper. Place the beetroot wedges alongside (or scatter them on top). Serve with the salad greens or spinach leaves alongside. Drizzle with balsamic vinegar.

The Food Effect Greek Salad

This protein-packed, fibre-filled salad is as good for you as it is colourful and delicious. What's more, with not much to do besides chopping some veg, it couldn't be easier to prepare.

Serves 2

2 large handfuls romaine lettuce, chopped
1 large or 2 small tomatoes, coarsely chopped
½ cucumber, coarsely diced
¼ small red onion, finely chopped
2 sticks of celery, sliced
80g reduced-fat feta cheese
32g pitted black olives

Dressing
2 tbsp olive oil
2 tsp lemon juice
1 garlic clove, crushed
½ tsp dried oregano
½ tsp dried dill
Salt and pepper, to taste

To make the dressing, whisk the olive oil, lemon juice, crushed garlic and herbs together until well blended. Season generously with salt and pepper. Combine all the salad ingredients, apart from the cheese and olives, in a large bowl. Add the dressing and toss through to coat. Top with the feta cheese and olives.

The Food Effect Skinny Chicken Salad Deluxe

This satisfying salad is great for those who want to lose weight without compromising on enjoying delicious meals.

Serves 1

150g skinless boneless chicken breast
Cajun spice, salt and pepper, to season chicken
2 handfuls mixed salad greens
½ cucumber, sliced
½ ripe avocado
10 cherry tomatoes
25g grated carrot
1 spring onion, sliced
Handful of mixed seeds

Dressing
3 tbsp light mayonnaise
1 tsp agave syrup

½ tsp whole-grain mustard
Water to thin, as needed

Dust the chicken breast with the Cajun spice, salt and pepper. Place it on a small baking tray and bake in a preheated oven to 180°C/Gas 4 oven for 20–25 minutes until cooked through. Once cooked, cut the chicken into strips. Arrange the salad greens in a bowl, place the grated carrots on top and arrange the tomatoes, spring onions and cucumber around. Cut the avocado into thin slices and place on top, along with chicken strips. Top with the mixed seeds.

For the dressing, thoroughly mix all the dressing ingredients together in a bowl. Serve in a bowl alongside the salad or drizzled over the top just before serving.

Chinese Chicken Stir-fry

Don't feel you need to serve hot vegetables with this dish – a fresh green salad complements it very well.

Serves 1

Spray cooking oil
100g skinless boneless chicken breast, cut into thin strips
1 tbsp low sodium soya sauce
½ fresh chilli, finely sliced, or ¼ tsp chilli powder
¼ tsp fresh ginger, grated, or a pinch of ground ginger
100g sugar snap peas, cut in halves crosswise
125g cooked brown rice, to serve

Spray a frying pan with cooking spray oil and heat over a medium-high heat. Once hot, add the chicken strips and stir-fry until cooked through (around 2–3 minutes). Add the soya sauce, fresh chilli or chilli powder, ginger and sugar snap peas. Cook for a further 2 minutes. Serve immediately with the brown rice and a fresh green salad.

Turkey-stuffed Peppers

This recipe can easily be doubled to make two portions.

Serves 1

1 onion, chopped
1 clove of garlic, crushed
100g lean turkey mince
200g tin chopped tomatoes
Handful of fresh spinach leaves
½ tsp salt
Black pepper to taste
¼ tsp turmeric
1 red pepper, top removed, cored and deseeded

Preheat the oven to 180°C/Gas 4. Spray a pan with cooking spray, add the onion and garlic and fry until the onion is translucent. Add the turkey mince and cook until the meat is no longer pink. Add the chopped tomatoes and spinach, stir well and cook until the spinach leaves wilt, about 3 minutes and add the salt, pepper and turmeric.

Using a small spoon, fill the red pepper with the turkey mixture. Place the pepper upright in a small baking dish. Bake for 30 minutes until the pepper has softened. Serve with a fresh green salad.

Spinach Salad with Strawberries

Serves 1

2 large handfuls baby spinach
1 large handful shredded romaine lettuce
75g strawberries, hulled and sliced
1 tbsp sunflower seeds

90g broccoli florets, chopped
1 hard-boiled egg, quartered
40g red kidney beans

Dressing
1 tbsp olive oil
2 tbsp balsamic vinegar
Salt and pepper, to taste

Combine all the salad ingredients. Mix together the olive oil and balsamic vinegar. Drizzle over the salad. Season with salt and pepper, and toss through.

Avocado and Almond Salad

Serves 1

1 tsp Dijon mustard
1 tbsp balsamic vinegar
Salt and pepper
2 large handfuls fresh spinach leaves
½ medium avocado, peeled and sliced
2 tbsp flaked almonds (toasted if desired)
1 tbsp dried cranberries

Mix together the mustard and balsamic vinegar, add salt and pepper, and mix well. Fill a plate or bowl with the spinach leaves, add the sliced avocado, and top with the flaked almonds and dried cranberries. Drizzle with the dressing, and adjust the seasoning to taste.

Cajun Chicken Breast with Red Cabbage Slaw

Serve with a fresh green salad and some brown rice or quinoa.

Serves 4

4 skinless, boneless chicken breasts (150–200g each)
2 tbsp lemon juice
2 tbsp olive oil
1 tsp chilli powder
½ tsp cumin
½ tsp dried coriander
½ tsp paprika
½ tsp dried basil
2 cloves of garlic, crushed
Salt and pepper

Red Cabbage Slaw
200g red cabbage, core removed
120ml apple cider or malt vinegar
4 tbsp agave syrup
2 tsp salt

Season the chicken well with salt and pepper. Combine the lemon juice, olive oil, seasonings and crushed garlic in a small mixing bowl or glass. Pour over the chicken, ensuring that both sides are well coated, and allow to marinate for at least 1 hour at room temperature, or overnight (up to twenty-four hours) in the fridge.

Shred the cabbage very finely using a food processor or sharp knife. Tip into a large bowl. Mix together the vinegar, agave syrup and salt until well combined. Pour over the cabbage; mix well. Set aside and allow to 'sit' for at least 1 hour before serving. Mix well before serving with the chicken.

Preheat the oven to 180°C/Gas 4. Arrange the marinated chicken in a single layer on a baking tray or ovenware dish that has been lightly coated with olive oil or spray oil. Pour the marinade over the chicken. Bake uncovered for about 20–30 minutes – do not overcook.

Cajun Chicken Breast Pitta

This is an easy, healthy and delicious way to use leftover Cajun Chicken (see page 214).

Serves 1

1 cooked Cajun Chicken Breast (see recipe)
1 whole-wheat pitta
2 tbsp mustard
1 tbsp reduced-sugar ketchup
Salad greens, sliced cucumber, tomatoes and red pepper

Use warm or cold cooked chicken breast – slice thinly on the diagonal. Cut the pitta bread in half. Spread inside of each half pitta with mustard and ketchup. Fill with salad greens, cucumber, tomatoes, red pepper and sliced chicken.

Healthy Hearty Minestrone

This versatile plant-based soup is low in fat, high in fibre and packed with vitamins, minerals and nutrients. The protein-packed beans and barley and satiety-promoting fibre, combined with nutrient-rich veggies and tomato broth (high in the super anti-oxidant lycopene) means this soup will fill you up not out!

Serves 6

2 tbsp olive oil
1 small onion, chopped
2 cloves of garlic, crushed
2 celery sticks (or additional courgettes), diced
1.9L vegetable stock (MSG-free)
400g tin cannellini beans
100g uncooked barley
4 carrots, diced
2 courgettes, diced
1 tsp dried basil
1 tsp dried oregano
1 tsp salt
¼ tsp black pepper
450g tinned chopped tomatoes
Crusty bread and Parmesan cheese, to serve (optional)

Heat the oil in a large pot over a medium heat. Add the onion, garlic and celery. Let them sauté until translucent, then pour in the stock, beans and barley. Simmer for 1 hour. Add the carrots, courgettes, herbs, salt and pepper. Simmer, uncovered, for a further hour. Add the tinned tomatoes and simmer for 20–30 minutes. Serve with the crusty bread and a sprinkling of Parmesan cheese.

Hummus Chicken

This is perfect served with brown rice and a mixed green salad, or chopped cucumber and tomato salad.

Serves 2

2 skinless, boneless chicken breasts (150g each)
120g reduced-fat hummus (store-bought or home-made, as recipe, below)

1 lemon, sliced into rounds, then halved
4 fresh rosemary sprigs or 2 tbsp dried rosemary
Generous drizzle of balsamic vinegar
Sea salt and freshly ground pepper

Hummus
400g tin chickpeas, drained and rinsed
1 clove of garlic
60g tahini
Juice of 1 lemon or 2 tbsp lemon juice
2 tbsp extra-virgin olive oil
1–2 tbsp water (adjust according to consistency)
1 tsp fine sea salt
¾ tsp ground cumin
¼ tsp black pepper

Preheat the oven to 200°C/Gas 6. Blend all the hummus ingredients together in a food processor (if making your own).

Place the chicken breasts in a small roasting pan and, using a spoon (or your hands), cover all the exposed chicken with the hummus, making sure that it's layered quite thickly. Scrunch each lemon half in your hand, then loosely arrange the lemon over the chicken with the rosemary sprigs, broken into smaller pieces. Season well with salt and pepper and drizzle with vinegar. Bake for about 20 minutes, until cooked through.

Protein-packed Pasta Dish

Serves 4 as a lunch or light supper

300g (raw weight) fusilli-shaped whole-wheat or brown rice pasta
1 courgette, thinly sliced and halved
1 red pepper, deseeded and diced
2 large vine tomatoes, cut into chunks

400g tin chickpeas, drained and rinsed
80g sliced black olives

Dressing
3 tbsp apple cider vinegar
1 tsp salt
1 tbsp mustard
3 cloves of garlic, crushed
3 tbsp olive oil
Pinch of cayenne pepper (optional but recommended)

Cook the pasta according to the packet directions. Drain and set aside. In a small jar, combine all the dressing ingredients and shake well. Place the cooked pasta, prepared vegetables, chickpeas and olives in a large bowl. Toss with the dressing and allow time for it to 'stand' (for the flavours to mingle) before serving. Serve at room temperature, or refrigerate and serve cold. Any leftovers make a great lunch the next day.

Vegetable Bolognaise

A healthy, delicious vegetarian version of the classic favourite, spaghetti bolognaise.

Serves 4

300g (dry weight) whole-wheat or brown rice spaghetti
1 tbsp olive oil
1 onion, chopped
2 carrots, peeled and finely chopped
2 sticks of celery, sliced
300g tin cut green beans in water, drained and chopped
400g tin chopped tomatoes
2 tbsp tomato purée
125g mushrooms, chopped

¼–½ tsp cayenne pepper
Salt and pepper
10g fresh parsley, chopped

Bring a large pot of water to the boil. Add a generous pinch of salt and stir. Add the spaghetti and cook according to the packet instructions.

In the meantime, heat the olive oil in a saucepan. Add the chopped onion and fry over a low heat for 3–5 minutes, until softened and translucent but not browned. Add the carrots, celery and green beans. Stir in the chopped tomatoes, tomato purée, mushrooms and cayenne pepper. Add a generous pinch of salt and pepper to taste. Allow to simmer for 10 minutes. Stir through the fresh parsley.

Drain the spaghetti when cooked, and divide between serving plates. Top each serving with a quarter of the bolognaise sauce. Top with some freshly ground black pepper. Serve hot.

Curried Chicken Salad

This recipe serves one if eaten alone as a main meal with salad greens; two if used to fill a sandwich or with rice, for example.

Serves 1–2

150g cooked chicken breast (skin removed), diced or shredded
2 spring onions, sliced thinly
1 celery stalk, finely diced
1 small tin of sweetcorn (150g), drained, or 1 large carrot, grated
2 tbsp raisins or dried cherries (optional)

Curry dressing
6 tbsp light mayonnaise
1 tbsp mustard
½ tsp curry powder
1 tbsp agave syrup or honey

1 tsp lemon juice
Generous pinch of salt
¼ tsp black pepper

Combine the dressing ingredients and stir together well. Put all the other ingredients in a mixing bowl, add the curry dressing and mix together until everything is well combined. Season with additional salt and pepper to taste.

Salmon and Sweet Potato Sliders with Roasted Red Pepper Sauce

A light twist on a classic favourite, these scrumptious salmon sliders are a fun mix of fishcake and salmon 'burger'. They're given a healthy makeover simply by baking instead of frying and using unadulterated sweet potato for extra bulk (and nutrients). Serve with the delicious Roasted Red Pepper Sauce opposite or simply enjoy them with a dollop of ketchup – despite what you may have heard, it's actually incredibly healthy and packed full of the antioxidant lycopene.

Makes 10–12 sliders

500g sweet potatoes
420g tinned red salmon (I use one large 418g tin), drained, skin removed
1 egg
1 tbsp lemon juice
½ tsp salt
¼ tsp black pepper
1 tsp dried dill
Lemon wedges
Roasted Red Pepper Sauce opposite, and/or ketchup, to serve

Peel the sweet potatoes and cut into small chunks. Place in a pot filled with water and bring to the boil. Simmer for about 15–20 minutes, until the potatoes are soft. Drain and allow to cool.

Place the cooked sweet potato, salmon (along with the bones – they're packed full of calcium), egg, lemon juice, salt, pepper and dill in a blender or food processor, and pulse until well combined and smooth. Refrigerate the mixture for at least 30 minutes.

Preheat the oven to 180°C/Gas 4. Line 2 baking trays with baking paper. Shape the mixture into 10–12 round 'sliders' on your prepared baking trays. Bake in the oven for 20–25 minutes. Serve warm or at room temperature, with the lemon wedges and Roasted Red Pepper Sauce or ketchup.

Roasted Red Pepper Sauce

Serve with Salmon and Sweet Potato Sliders (see above), or with any fish, chicken or vegetarian dish (such as falafel balls and salads). This sauce keeps well for several days in the fridge, and is also delicious with freshly cut vegetable sticks.

70g roasted red peppers from jar, drained (or roast your own, using 2 red peppers)
120g light mayonnaise
1 clove of garlic, peeled
1 tbsp lemon juice
½ tsp salt
¼ tsp black pepper

Combine all the ingredients in a food processor and blend until completely smooth. Store in the fridge.

Eggs in a Mug

Serve this simple dish with fresh vegetables and whole-grain crackers or toast.

Serves 1

Non-stick cooking spray
2 eggs
Skimmed, soya or almond milk
Pinch of salt
1 large handful fresh spinach leaves, torn

Spray a microwave-safe mug with non-stick cooking spray. Crack the 2 eggs into a bowl. Add a dash of milk, a pinch of salt and the torn-up spinach leaves. Mix the ingredients together well with a fork. Pour into the prepared mug and put it in the microwave for about 1 minute 50 seconds on high. If the mixture has not set or is still raw after this time, cook for a few more seconds. Allow a few minutes for the dish to set and cool, then put on a plate to serve.

Saucy Salmon and Veggie Bake

I created this recipe to provide a healthy, protein-packed one-pot meal that's easy to whip up, and is great for a filling fancy lunch or a delicious week-night dinner.

Serves 4

2 red onions, skinned and cut into wedges
2 red peppers, deseeded and cut into 2cm squares
2 medium courgettes, cut into 2cm slices
4 small sweet potatoes, peeled and cut into 1cm slices
1 tbsp olive oil
4 salmon fillets (150g each)
Fresh chives, to serve (optional)

Sauce
5 tbsp passata or finely chopped tomatoes (you can use tinned)
1 tbsp soya sauce
1 tbsp agave syrup
1 tbsp apple cider vinegar
Salt and pepper

Mix together the sauce ingredients and season with salt and pepper, according to taste. Preheat the oven to 200°C/Gas 6. Line a large baking sheet with foil. Place the prepared vegetables in a large bowl with the oil and toss to coat.

Place the vegetables in a single layer on the baking sheet and roast in the oven for 30 minutes. Remove the baking sheet from the oven, and put the cooked vegetables in a medium-sized roasting dish. Dip each piece of salmon in the prepared sauce to coat. Tip any remaining sauce over the vegetables and mix. Place the coated salmon fillets on top of the vegetables. Put the roasting pan in the preheated oven. Bake for 15–20 minutes. Garnish with the fresh chives to serve.

Tuscan-style Tuna Bean Salad

This is my version of a popular Italian dish. The combination of lean protein in the tuna, fibre in the beans (plus more protein) and antioxidant-rich tomatoes, make it an ideal Food Effect-friendly meal.

Serves 4

2 x 150–170g tins tuna in oil*
2 large or 4 small vine tomatoes, sliced into rings
Sea salt and black pepper
1 bunch spring onions, chopped
1 small handful fresh basil leaves, roughly torn
400g tin cannellini beans, drained and rinsed
Fresh chopped flat-leaf parsley

Dressing
2 tbsp balsamic vinegar
2 tbsp extra-virgin olive oil
Salt and pepper, to taste

Place the tuna in a large bowl and break up with a fork. Layer the ingredients in the order listed (beginning with the tomatoes, and ending with the parsley to garnish) in a large serving bowl. Mix together the vinegar and oil and drizzle over the tuna mixture. Season generously with sea salt and black pepper. Allow to stand for at least 30 minutes before serving. Toss through before serving.

*While I normally advocate tuna in water or brine throughout The Food Effect diet, that's factoring in the addition of some mayonnaise in almost all The Food Effect meal options. This recipe doesn't include any mayonnaise, and using tuna in oil is essential for the recipe. Additionally, the sunflower oil in tinned tuna is heart healthy, and it doesn't add any unhealthy or unnecessary calories – so don't try to substitute the tinned tuna in oil with dry tuna.

SOUPS AND SIDE DISHES

Here are two fantastic low-carb, low-calorie highly nutritious recipes for 'miraculous mash'. As I'm sure you'll know by now, I'm not a fan of cutting out carbs, but these comforting bowls of goodness provide far more goodness and far fewer calories than a big bowl of white potatoes. And of course the taste is nothing less than miraculous!

Miraculous Cauliflower Mash

Serves 4

600g frozen cauliflower
2 cloves of garlic, peeled and sliced

1 tsp salt
1–2 tbsp milk or soya milk
Black pepper, to taste

Boil the cauliflower and garlic in a large pot of boiling water until soft (about 20 minutes). Drain completely. Transfer the cauliflower and garlic to a large bowl, add salt and purée using a hand-held blender (or use a food processor) until completely smooth and 'whipped'. Add the milk as necessary, and blend again to achieve the desired mash consistency (don't allow it to get too thin). Season with black pepper to taste.

Miraculous Butternut Squash Mash

Serves 4

1 large butternut squash (1–1.5kg), peeled*, seeded and cubed
1 tsp salt
½ tsp cinnamon
2 tbsp agave or maple syrup, or honey
Chopped pecan nuts or walnuts for garnish (optional)

*Tip for peeling butternut squash with ease. Place whole, uncooked butternut in 180°C/Gas 4 oven for 30 minutes. Remove and allow to cool until manageable, then peel. Doing this makes the peeling process so much easier.

Fill a large saucepan with enough water to cover the butternut squash. Bring to a boil over a medium heat. Add the squash cubes. Reduce the heat, cover and simmer for about 30 minutes, or until the squash is completely soft and tender. Drain, and transfer to a bowl. Add the salt, cinnamon and agave or maple syrup, and blend with a hand-held blender (or use a food processor) until completely smooth. Serve warm, garnished with the chopped pecan nuts or walnuts, and cinnamon and syrup if desired.

The Food Effect World Cup Pea Soup

This creamy yet light and refreshing soup recipe was born out of a dinner party I organised without realising the timing clashed with the football World Cup final. Thankfully, it was a great success, with guests proclaiming it one of the best soups they'd ever tasted (one football fanatic even said it was worth missing the final for). I serve it with fresh seeded bread and top it with pumpkin seeds but you could also try some of the other suggestions outlined below.

Serves 4–6

2 tbsp olive oil
1 large onion, chopped
800ml chicken or vegetable stock (made from MSG-free powder or liquid stock)
15g fresh mint leaves
800g frozen peas
1 head of romaine or cos lettuce, torn into shreds
2 tsp fine sea salt
½ tsp black pepper
Pumpkin seeds/toasted chopped cashew nuts/chopped chives/mint leaves, to garnish

Heat the oil in a large pot and gently fry the chopped onion until clear and softened. Add the stock and stir in the mint leaves and peas. Bring to the boil and simmer for 15 minutes. Add the lettuce, salt and pepper. Simmer for another 10 minutes.

Purée the soup well, using a hand-held blender, until smooth and thick. Serve hot, garnished with the seeds, nuts or herbs.

Easiest Ever Red Lentil Soup

Quick, easy, healthy and delicious, this one-pot recipe almost cooks itself and doesn't require blending.

Serves 4–6

2 tsp olive oil
1 onion, chopped
2 cloves of garlic, crushed
1 tsp ground cumin
300g red lentils, rinsed
1.4L chicken or vegetable stock (made from MSG-free powder or liquid stock)
Salt and pepper to taste
2 tbsp lemon juice
Fresh coriander, to serve (optional)

Heat the oil in a medium-sized pot, add the chopped onion and garlic and cook for 3–5 minutes until softened. Add the cumin and cook for 1 minute. Stir in the lentils and mix well. Add the stock, salt and pepper, and bring to a boil. Reduce the heat, cover and simmer until the lentils are soft and tender, and the soup is beginning to thicken (about 30–40 minutes). Add the lemon juice and stir through well. Adjust the seasoning by adding salt and pepper according to taste. Serve sprinkled with fresh chopped coriander if desired.

Carrot, Ginger and Sweet Potato Soup

Serves 4

1 large onion, chopped
1 tbsp peeled, chopped fresh ginger
1 tbsp coconut oil

7 medium-sized carrots, peeled and thickly sliced
1 large sweet potato, peeled and cubed
1L chicken or vegetable stock (made from MSG-free powder or liquid stock)
Salt and pepper, to taste
Chopped fresh coriander, red pepper or chilli flakes, pumpkin seeds or toasted flaked almonds, to garnish (optional)

In a large pot, sauté the onion and ginger in the oil until transparent. Add the carrots and sweet potato, and cook over a low heat until slightly tender. Stir in the stock. Bring to a boil. Reduce the heat, cover and simmer for 30–40 minutes. Once fully cooked, turn off the heat and blend the soup until completely smooth, using a hand-held immersion blender. Add salt and pepper to taste.

Serve sprinkled with any of the garnishes outlined above.

Gorgeously Green Soup

As gorgeous in taste, texture and appearance as it is good for you!

Serves 2

1 tbsp olive oil
1 small onion, diced
1 clove of garlic, crushed
180g fresh spinach leaves
300g tinned baby carrots, drained
360ml hot vegetable stock (made from MSG-free powder or liquid stock)
½ tsp salt
2 thick brown rice cakes

Heat the oil in a large pot over a medium heat. Add the onion and garlic and cook for about 3–5 minutes until the onion is soft and translucent. Add the spinach leaves, carrots, hot stock and salt. Stir together and simmer for about 5 minutes until the spinach leaves have wilted. Turn off the heat and add the rice cakes by crumbling them in. Stir well. Leave for several minutes to go soggy. Purée the soup with a hand-held blender until well combined and completely smooth.

Fresh Tomato Soup with Mixed Green Pesto

Low in fat and deliciously satisfying, this soup is full of fibre, vitamins and antioxidants. The addition of fresh spinach and basil pesto gives extra flavor, as well as a wealth of nutritional goodness.

Serves 4

1½kg large ripe tomatoes
2 tbsp olive oil
1 tsp dry oregano
Salt and pepper to taste
1 onion, chopped
2 cloves of garlic, crushed
1 large carrot, diced
1 stick of celery, chopped
480ml vegetable stock (made from MSG-free powder or liquid stock)
2 tsp tomato purée
1 tsp stevia or xylitol

Pesto
100g fresh baby spinach leaves
100g fresh basil leaves
120g walnuts
2 cloves of garlic
½–1 tsp sea salt, to taste
5 tbsp olive oil

First make the soup. Preheat the oven to 200°C/Gas 6. Cut the tomatoes horizontally and place them cut-side up on a parchment-lined baking tray. Drizzle with oil, sprinkle with the oregano, and season with salt and pepper. Place in the oven and bake until the tomatoes are soft and a bit charred (about 45 minutes). Meanwhile, heat 2 tablespoons of oil over a medium heat in a large pan and add the onion, garlic, carrot and celery. Cook, stirring regularly, for about 6 minutes until softened. Add the baked tomatoes and all the juices from the baking tray to the onion mixture, together with the vegetable stock and tomato purée. Simmer for about 30 minutes until all the vegetables are soft. Allow to cool a little, then purée the soup until smooth, using a hand-held blender. Season to taste with salt and pepper. Serve the soup drizzled with the pesto.

To make the pesto, purée the spinach, basil, nuts, garlic and salt in a blender, then slowly add the oil to make a smooth paste. Add a bit of water if too thick. (Pesto can be frozen in ice-cube trays and used when needed.)

Winning Combo Salad

This vibrant, nutrient-packed salad is colourful, eye-catching and delicious.

Serves 4

200g raw beetroot, grated
2 large carrots, grated
1 large tin (340g) of corn, drained
300g frozen peas, thawed

Dressing
2 large ripe tomatoes
2 tbsp agave syrup or honey
4 tbsp extra-virgin olive oil

1 tbsp soya sauce
Salt and pepper to taste

Combine all the salad ingredients in a large bowl. Blend the dressing ingredients together in a food processor or using a hand-held blender. Pour over the salad and toss through well. Adjust the seasoning to taste. Cover and refrigerate until ready to serve.

Red Cabbage Slaw

Serves 4

200g red cabbage, core removed
120ml apple cider or malt vinegar
4 tbsp agave syrup
2 tsp salt

Shred the cabbage very finely using a food processor or sharp knife. Tip into a large bowl. Mix together the vinegar, agave syrup and salt until well combined. Pour over the cabbage and mix well. Set aside and allow to 'stand' for at least 1 hour before serving. Mix again well before serving.

Quinoa Salad with Avocado, Mango and Pomegranate

An incredibly versatile recipe, this salad can be served alongside grilled chicken or fish but is also substantial enough to make a delicious light lunch or dinner. If you'd like to add some additional protein and flavour, top it with some feta, halloumi or goats' cheese.

Serves 2 as a main course, 4 as a side dish

170g uncooked red quinoa (or regular white quinoa)
1 ripe avocado, diced
1 small ripe mango, peeled and diced
80g pomegranate seeds
20g pistachio nuts, shelled
4 spring onions, thinly sliced
A few handfuls of spinach or salad leaves

Dressing
1 tbsp olive oil
2 tbsp balsamic vinegar
1 tsp sesame oil

Cook the quinoa according to the packet instructions. Allow to cool slightly. Put all the salad ingredients in a large bowl. Whisk together the dressing ingredients. Add to the salad, and toss well to coat.

Rainbow Brown Rice Salad

This colourful, substantial salad is guaranteed to go down a treat on any buffet table. Leftovers also make a great packed lunch, along with some salad greens. This dish is low in fat, high in fibre and full of vitamins, minerals and protein.

Serves 8 as a side dish

50g cashew nuts
6 tbsp mixed seeds (such as sunflower, pumpkin and sesame seeds)
450g uncooked brown rice
1 tsp salt
6 spring onions, thinly sliced (green tops removed and discarded)
1 red pepper, deseeded and diced
1 orange pepper, deseeded and diced
60g currants or raisins

3 tbsp fresh parsley, chopped
325g tin sweetcorn, drained

Dressing
2 tbsp sunflower oil
6 tbsp soya sauce
2 tbsp lemon juice
1 large clove of garlic, crushed
Generous pinch of sea salt
¼ tsp black pepper
½ tsp ground ginger or fresh ginger, peeled and finely chopped
½ tsp chilli powder (optional)

Place all the dressing ingredients in a sealable jar, and shake well.
Toast the cashew nuts and mixed seeds in a preheated 180°C/Gas 4
oven until golden (keep a good eye on them, as they burn quickly),
and allow to cool. (This step can be done in advance, and the nut
mixture can then be stored in an airtight container or Ziplock bag.)

Cook the rice in 950ml of boiling water with salt for about 40 minutes, until the water is fully absorbed and the rice is soft and cooked.
Drain and add the dressing to the rice while the rice is still warm. Stir
through. Transfer to a serving bowl and allow to cool completely. Add
all the remaining ingredients to the rice at least 1 hour before serving.
Mix well. Serve either at room temperature, or chilled from the fridge.

Quinoa Tabbouleh Salad

It is delicious as a side dish with fish or chicken, or topped with feta
cheese, olives and avocado for a delicious light lunch or dinner.

Serves 4 as a side dish

480ml water
½ tsp salt

170g uncooked quinoa
2 medium tomatoes, diced
1 small cucumber, diced
½ small red onion, finely chopped
40g fresh flat-leaf parsley, finely chopped
Juice of 1 lemon (2 tbsp lemon juice)
60ml olive oil
Salt and pepper to taste

Bring the water to a boil over a low heat, with the ½ tsp salt and quinoa. Cover and simmer gently for 15–20 minutes until the grains are cooked but still a little firm. Remove from the heat and allow to cool. Add the chopped tomatoes, cucumber, red onion and parsley. Dress with the lemon juice and olive oil, and season generously with salt and pepper. Toss together well. Chill and either serve cold from the fridge or allow to come up to room temperature.

SNACKS AND SWEET TREATS

Healthy Home-made Peanut Butter

This is an all-natural alternative to store-bought peanut butter.

Makes 1 large jar

450g roasted peanuts (without skins)
Generous pinch of sea salt (omit if using salted peanuts)
1–2 tbsp agave syrup

Put the ingredients in the bowl of a food processor. Process until the nuts break down to form a completely smooth, creamy, peanut butter consistency, stopping at intervals to scrape down the sides of the processor. This process does take some time (about 10 minutes, depending on the power of your processor), so do be patient and don't think it hasn't worked – the nuts go from crushed, to fine crumbs, to a course dough-ball, but then eventually break down to a perfect peanut butter consistency.

Once completely smooth, pour into a sealable jar and store in the fridge for several weeks – if it lasts that long!

Best-ever Healthy Home-made Hummus

The quantities of ingredients here make quite a small batch. I always double them if making the hummus for guests (or for the week), and recommend doing so. Leftovers never go to waste.

Serves 4

400g tin chickpeas, drained and rinsed
1 clove of garlic
60g tahini
Juice of 1 lemon
1 tsp fine sea salt
¾ tsp ground cumin
¼ tsp black pepper
2 tbsp extra-virgin olive oil
1–2 tbsp water (adjust according to consistency)

Place the chickpeas, garlic, tahini, lemon juice, salt, cumin and pepper in the bowl of a food processor fitted with a metal blade. Process for 1 minute until fully blended. Add the olive oil and 1 tbsp water, then process again until fully combined and smooth. Add the additional 1 tbsp water if a thinner consistency of hummus is desired, and blend. (The recipe can also be made in a blender, or using a hand-held blender with the ingredients placed in a large mixing bowl.) Transfer the hummus to an airtight container and store in the fridge.

Serve with whole-wheat pitta, crackers or crudités, or simply eat it and enjoy it as is.

Flourless Peanut Butter Biscuits

A long-time favourite recipe of mine, and boasting just three main ingredients, these cookies couldn't possibly be more delicious ... or easier to make.

Makes 12–15 biscuits

250g natural peanut butter (smooth or crunchy)
250g coconut sugar
1 egg
½ tsp vanilla extract
¼–½ tsp salt (¼ tsp if peanut butter is already salted, ½ tsp if using unsalted)
Dark chocolate chips or chopped roasted salted peanuts (optional)
Fine sea salt

Preheat the oven to 180°C/Gas 4. Line 2 baking trays with baking paper (do not grease or spray with oil). Place all the ingredients (apart from the optional add-ins) in a medium-sized mixing bowl. Using an electric hand beater or beating by hand with a spoon, mix until every-thing is completely combined to form a dough. If using chocolate chips or chopped peanuts, add them and mix through at this point.

Form the dough into balls (each measuring 2 level tbsp dough) and place on the prepared baking trays. Press down on each ball very lightly with the back of a fork (see note below).

Bake for 10–12 minutes or until just browned. Sprinkle a small amount of fine sea salt onto each biscuit when the biscuits come out of the oven. Allow to cool for 5 minutes on the baking tray, before transferring to a wire rack to cool completely.

Note If you like a crispier, more 'classic'-style, flatter biscuit, flatten the dough slightly before baking (this will cause the biscuits to spread more). If you prefer a softer, more dense biscuit (as I do), leave the dough in balls and do not flatten them at all; once they come out of the oven, flatten them slightly with the back of a fork, then allow to cool (this will achieve a 'biscuit' shape, with a more dense and compact texture).

All-healthy Raw Chocolate Truffle Balls

These truffle balls freeze well and are one of my all-time favourites. I like to keep a batch in stock so that I always have healthy snacks at hand.

Makes 15–18 balls

265g pitted Medjool dates (soak dates in hot water for 10–20 minutes if they are not soft)
25g unsweetened cocoa powder
70g unsalted almonds
70g walnuts or peanuts
¼ tsp salt
2 tsp vanilla extract
75g desiccated coconut (for rolling) and/or goji berries to decorate (optional)

Put all the ingredients (excluding the coconut) in a food processor. Blend for a few minutes until a thick 'dough' is formed (but still keeps some fine texture from the nuts). Keep scraping down the sides of the processor to incorporate all the dry ingredients. Transfer the mixture to a bowl. Scoop into 1 heaped tablespoon-sized portions and roll into smooth balls with your hands. If using, place the coconut (or any desired topping) in a shallow bowl, and roll the moist dough balls in it to fully cover them. Place in the fridge for at least 30 minutes before serving.

Raw Bakewell Tart Balls

These balls freeze well and are perfect to have at hand for healthy snacking. They taste so good it's hard to believe they're all-natural and good for you too!

Makes 15–18 balls

150g unsalted cashew nuts
175g pitted Medjool dates
40g raisins
40g dried cranberries
½ tsp vanilla extract or essence
½ tsp almond essence
¼ tsp salt

Put all the ingredients in a food processor. Blend for a few minutes until a thick 'dough' is formed (which still keeps some fine texture from the nuts). Keep scraping down the sides of the processor to incorporate all the dry ingredients. Transfer the mixture to a bowl. Scoop into 1 heaped tablespoon-sized portions, and roll into smooth balls using your hands. Place in the fridge for at least 30 minutes before serving.

Sweet and Healthy Hummus Muffins

These high-fibre, protein-packed muffins are soft, sweet and delicious.

Makes 6–8 muffins

1 large apple, peeled, cored and roughly chopped
120g hummus
80ml agave syrup or honey
2 eggs
1 tbsp vanilla extract

2 tbsp ground almonds or almond flour (or wholemeal flour)
1 tsp bicarbonate of soda
1 tbsp ground cinnamon
½ tsp salt
50g roughly chopped prunes, Medjool dates or raisins

Preheat the oven to 180°C/Gas 4. In a food processor, combine the apple and hummus, and pulse until well blended. Add the agave syrup or honey, eggs, vanilla, ground almonds, bicarbonate of soda, cinnamon and salt, and pulse to combine. Pour the batter into a greased muffin tray (or one lined with paper or silicone cases), and fill each until three-quarters full. Bake for 20 minutes, until firm to the touch on top and a toothpick inserted into a muffin comes out clean. Allow to cool. The muffins can be stored in an airtight container or Ziploc bag for several days, or they can be frozen to be enjoyed whenever you fancy.

Chocolate Peanut Clusters

Quick and easy to make, these 'no-bake' clusters require just a few ingredients. Delicious and not too naughty, they're perfect home-made treats.

12oz dark chocolate or dark chocolate chips
8oz roasted (salted) peanuts
Pinch of salt (if using unsalted peanuts)

Line a large baking tray with baking paper or foil and set aside. Melt the chocolate in a heavy-based pan over a low heat. Keep stirring, making sure you don't burn the chocolate. As soon as the chocolate has melted, turn off the heat. Add the peanuts to the melted chocolate and stir well until they are fully mixed in and coated. Spoon heaping tablespoons of the mixture onto the prepared baking tray. Allow to cool. Place in the fridge and allow to set for several hours. Remove from the baking paper or foil.

The Chocolate Peanut Clusters can be stored in an airtight container in the fridge or freezer for several weeks.

Fudgy Flourless Peanut Butter Hummus Bars

Boasting protein, healthy fats and fibre, these bars are a perfect option for a mid-afternoon snack paired with some fruit.

Makes 8 medium-sized bars

120g hummus (shop bought or home-made)
125g natural peanut butter (creamy or crunchy)
250g coconut sugar
1 large egg
½ tsp vanilla essence
½ tsp cinnamon
¼–½ tsp salt (¼ tsp if peanut butter is already salted, ½ tsp if using unsalted)

Put all the ingredients in a large bowl. Mix together well using a hand-held electric beater, until the mixture is smooth and well combined. Pour the batter into a small loaf tin lined with non-stick baking paper. Bake in a preheated 180°C/Gas 4 oven for about 25 minutes, until firm. Allow to cool completely then remove from the tin and cut into eight bars.

No-bake Fibre-filled Brownie Bars

Decadent, filling and delicious, it's hard to believe that these brownie bars are super-healthy, all-natural and perfect when you want something sweet but also want to stick to your healthy eating habits.

Makes 8 bars

115g unsalted almonds, cashew nuts or peanuts (or use a mixture)
20g unsweetened desiccated coconut
175g pitted Medjool dates
65g soft prunes
2 tbsp cocoa powder
¼ tsp salt
2–3 tbsp agave syrup, to taste

Blend the nuts in a food processor or blender until finely ground. Add the rest of the ingredients to the processor, and blend until well combined and a 'dough-like' mixture has formed. Line a small loaf tin with baking paper. Put the mixture in the tin, and press down firmly. Place in the fridge for several hours then remove from the tin and cut into squares or bars. Store in the fridge or freezer (allow time to defrost the bars when you want to eat them).

Peanut Cookie Energy Balls

Looking for the perfect snack to have on hand for those mid-afternoon munchies or late-night sweet cravings? These all-healthy energy balls are just the thing!

Makes 15–18 balls

140g roasted, salted peanuts
265g pitted dates
50g uncooked oats (use gluten-free if required)
1 tsp cinnamon
¼ tsp ground ginger (optional)
1 tsp vanilla essence
¼ tsp salt

Put all the ingredients in a food processor or blender. Blend for a few minutes until a thick 'dough' is formed. Keep scraping down the sides of the processor to get all the dry ingredients incorporated. Transfer the mixture to a bowl. Scoop into 1 heaped tablespoon-sized portions and roll into smooth balls with your hands. Put in the fridge for at least 30 minutes before serving.

Tropical Mango Energy Balls

These freeze well and make a great tropical-tasting snack.

Makes about 18 balls

150g unsalted cashew nuts
115g pitted Medjool dates
125g dried mango, soaked in mug of hot water for about 10–15 minutes, then drained
½ tsp vanilla essence
Pinch of ground turmeric
¼ tsp salt
Desiccated coconut, for rolling (optional, but recommended)

Put all the ingredients, except the coconut, if using, in a food processor or blender. Blend for a few minutes until a thick 'dough' is formed. Keep scraping down the sides of processor to get all the dry ingredients incorporated. Transfer the mixture to a bowl. Scoop into 1 heaped tablespoon-sized portions and roll into smooth balls using your hands. Roll in the desiccated coconut to coat (if desired). Put in the fridge for at least 30 minutes before serving.

Flourless Carrot Cake (Gluten-free, Dairy-free)

Carrot cake must be one of the most popular cakes for tea-time, as well as a personal favourite. This guilt-free version is made without flour or refined sugar but it definitely does not compromise on flavour! Although this cake is super-healthy, you'll still need to exercise some discipline and enjoy it in moderation. Stick to one slice, as indicated in the lifestyle-phase suggestions.

3 large eggs
200g coconut palm sugar (or light brown sugar)
2 tsp vanilla essence
120ml melted coconut oil
200g ground almonds
100g desiccated coconut
2 tsp cinnamon
½ tsp nutmeg
50g grated carrot
100g pecan nuts or walnuts, roughly chopped

Dairy-free icing (optional)
150g unsalted cashew nuts, soaked in boiling water for 30 minutes, or overnight in cold water
60ml agave or maple syrup
2 tbsp coconut oil
1 tsp vanilla extract
Pinch of sea salt

First make the cake. Preheat the oven to 160°C/Gas 3. Beat the eggs, sugar, vanilla and oil until light and well combined. Add the ground almonds, coconut, cinnamon and nutmeg, and stir until just combined. Then add the grated carrot and chopped nuts, and mix until well combined. Line a 23cm spring-form tin with baking paper and spray the sides with non-stick baking spray or oil. Spoon the batter into the prepared pan. Bake for 45 minutes to 1 hour, until a toothpick inserted in the cake comes out clean. Allow the cake to cool in the tin for about 10 minutes, then loosen the edges with a knife and remove from the tin to cool.

To make the icing, if using, drain and rinse the soaked cashew nuts.

Combine all the ingredients in a high-speed blender or food processor, and blend until smooth and creamy. You may need to scrape the mixture down and pulse a few times to achieve the desired consistency. Remove from the blender and set aside. Spread over the carrot cake once it has completely cooled.

CHAPTER 14

Kitchen Staples and Tips

To ensure your healthy-lifestyle changes last

Kitchen staples

Keep a selection of the following in your store cupboard, fridge and freezer, to ensure that healthy meals or snacks can always be put together in a matter of minutes. Of course, this is just a guide for you to use and adapt according to your own individual taste, preferences and lifestyle.

Fresh fruit and vegetables

- Apples
- Pears
- Oranges
- Blueberries
- Pre-cut carrot sticks (or whole carrots)
- Tomatoes, cherry tomatoes
- Cucumber
- Spinach, salad leaves
- Sweet potatoes
- Avocados

Whole grains

- Brown rice
- Lentils (such as dried red lentils)
- Quinoa
- Oats (such as porridge oats and rolled oats)
- Whole-wheat or brown rice pasta
- Whole-wheat couscous
- Wholemeal or rye bread
- Whole-wheat pitta bread
- Ryvita, brown rice cakes, oatcakes, Corn Thins

Nuts and seeds

- Almonds (whole)
- Flaked almonds
- Cashew nuts
- Walnuts
- Peanuts
- Pistachio nuts
- Desiccated coconut (unsweetened)
- Pumpkin seeds
- Sunflower seeds
- Sesame seeds
- Mixed seeds
- Peanut or almond butter

Dried fruit

- Raisins
- Dried apricots
- Prunes
- Dates

Tinned foods

- Chopped tomatoes
- Cannellini beans
- Chickpeas
- Corn
- Red kidney beans
- Lentils
- Peas
- Tuna (in water or brine)
- Salmon

Oils, vinegars and condiments

- Apple cider vinegar
- Balsamic vinegar
- Extra-virgin olive oil (for drizzling and dressings)
- Olive oil (for cooking)
- Coconut oil
- Soya sauce (reduced sodium/'Lite')
- Mustard
- Ketchup (Heinz: reduced salt and sugar)
- Lemon juice

Dried herbs and spices

- Cinnamon
- Cayenne pepper
- Chilli powder
- Coriander
- Cumin
- Curry powder
- Dill
- Ginger
- Garlic powder

- Paprika
- Turmeric
- Table salt and sea salt
- Black pepper

Sweeteners

- Agave syrup
- Honey
- Stevia or xylitol (granulated)
- Cinnamon
- Cocoa powder

Fridge

- Skimmed, soya and almond milks
- Low-fat cottage cheese
- Low-fat cream cheese
- Low-fat/fat-free natural yoghurts, fat-free Greek yoghurt (such as Total 0%)
- Eggs
- Hummus (reduced fat)

Freezer

- Sliced bread: wholemeal, rye
- Whole-wheat pitta
- Frozen broccoli
- Cauliflower
- Frozen green beans
- Frozen peas
- Corn, corn on the cob
- Vegetarian burgers (a natural brand such as Fry's)

Essential extras

- Herbal teas, green tea
- Coffee
- Nākd bars, Trek bars (these are all all-natural, not too high in calories and have a good protein content, with no added sugar or unhealthy fats)
- Dark chocolate (70 per cent cocoa or above)

A reminder of The Food Effect basics

While you may not immediately remember or follow every single thing I've recommended throughout this whole book (as the saying goes: 'Rome wasn't built in a day'), what I do strongly advise is that you follow and stick to from the start are The Food Effect fundamentals for healthy eating and weight loss and The Food Effect rules. Here they are as a reminder:

Eat whole, natural foods Avoid packaged, processed foods as much as possible. This means eating whole, natural foods that are close to, if not the same as, their natural state; for example, fresh fruit, vegetables, whole grains, nuts, eggs, dairy foods and fish. The shorter the list of ingredients on a package of food, the better it is.

Make sure you never get too hungry Long gaps between meals disrupt your blood-sugar levels, leading to excessive hunger, cravings and stress eating. When you do eventually eat, you will be so hungry that it will take a lot more food to feel satisfied, and it's unlikely that you'll binge on celery sticks. Eating small, healthy snacks between meals helps keep your blood sugar levels stable and your metabolism going strong. The suggested snacks in the attack phase (see page 175) and the list of snacks in the lifestyle phase meal options (see page 176) should help you with this.

Stay well hydrated Often when we think we're hungry, we're actually just thirsty. Water aids weight loss by keeping your cells functioning at their fat-burning best, and also helps your kidneys to flush out excess toxins and chemicals, which may be slowing down your metabolism. Make sure you drink plenty of water throughout the day, as well as 1–2 glasses *before* every meal or snack you have. See more on this on page 253.

Slow down your eating and enjoy your food Focus on the food you're eating and don't just wolf it down. Avoid eating dinner in front of the TV or lunch in front of your computer; take time out to enjoy your meal and actually pay attention to what you're having. This will also ensure that your brain actually registers when you've eaten enough food.

Eat healthy fats – don't go fat-free This means eating good, healthy unsaturated fats found in nuts, peanut butter, avocados, olive oil, and various other healthy oils. Incorporating good fats into your diet will help to reduce sugar cravings, increase energy levels and keep you fuller for longer. While too much fat can cause weight gain, too little of the right fats prevents your cells from functioning properly, which affects fat metabolism, hormone balance and energy – all leading to weight gain. There is more detailed information on fats in Chapter 6.

Don't shun carbs Instead, stick to whole-grain, unrefined carbohydrates such as oats, wholemeal or rye bread, brown rice, sweet potatoes and quinoa. Slow-release carbs from whole-grain sources will give you the get up and go you need to stay active and full of energy, while keeping your metabolism going strong and steady all day (and night). They are also great sources of fibre and various other essential nutrients.

Know yourself and be realistic Each individual has different needs, goals and preferences, combined with different body types and genetic make-up. You have to recognise your individual needs and be realistic about the changes you can make. For example, if you enjoy having your evening snack late at night, there's no point trying to force yourself to eat it earlier in the day. Evidence has refuted the myth that calories eaten late at night are 'worse', and has proven that a calorie is a calorie is a calorie. Whether you eat it at 7 p.m. or midnight, there's no difference; it's your overall daily consumption that counts, which is why you're allowed an evening treat every night.

Eat a rainbow Whether it's fresh, frozen or tinned – try to increase and vary your intake of fruit and vegetables. You'll feel so much better and your body will benefit from all the added vitamins, nutrients, antioxidants and fibre. Diets rich in fruit and vegetables have been proven to decrease the risk of heart attacks, strokes and a variety of cancers, while healthy, glowing skin is also achieved by eating a colourful, varied diet.

Know your portions Just because it's healthy, it doesn't mean it can't make you gain weight. Even if you stick to healthy foods, you still have to watch your portion sizes and quantities when consuming foods such as nuts, hummus, avocados, olive oil and dark chocolate (that is, all the things marked with an asterisk in the tables in Chapter 2). Just because they're healthy it does not mean that you can eat them freely. There's definitely benefit in consuming a little olive oil, but pouring it liberally over your pasta and dipping your bread in it will lead to excessive calories and weight gain. The same goes for nuts – learn what a normal serving size looks like (this is specified throughout the book), and limit yourself to that.

The Food Effect rules

Prepare, prepare, prepare This is the golden rule of healthy eating habits. The more planned and organised you are, the easier and more likely healthy eating and living will be. Pack your own lunch if possible, pre-chop vegetables to have on hand for meals and snacks, and keep your fridge and cupboards stocked with the right healthy foods as listed on pages 245–249.

Avoid highly processed and packaged foods as much as possible Read the labels on food products – don't buy what you can't pronounce or have never heard of.

Don't go hungry Never leave more than 3–4 hours without something small to eat. Always carry some healthy snacks with you if you know you're going to be out and about for a while or working long hours. For convenience, all snacks are listed in your plan and are super easy – so there's really no excuse.

But . . .

Don't go grazing Eating regularly does *not* mean you should be constantly picking throughout the day. The calories in a few nuts 'here and there' add up. Stick to your three meals and two snacks per day – and nothing outside of that. Have them whenever you feel it suits you, your schedule and your hunger levels best.

Ditch the white stuff Cutting out the white stuff is one of the easiest ways to lose weight and improve your health. Most processed, refined foods (think sugar, white bread, flour, pasta and sugary low-fibre cereals – *not* egg whites, cauliflower and white fish) are just empty calories with little fibre and goodness.

But don't cut out all starchy foods As explained in Chapter 3, that's a recipe for a long-term 'diet disaster'.

Eat good fats As outlined in Chapter 6, you need some good fat to burn fat. This means eating healthy unsaturated fats found in nuts, peanut butter and avocados, olive oil, and various other healthy oils. These are all included (in specified amounts) in the plan, as they have been proved to lower the risk of heart disease and aid the body in the absorption of vitamins and minerals, as well as helping with satiety, cravings and weight loss.

Avoid trans-fats Often listed under the names 'hydrogenated oil' or 'hydrogenated vegetable fat' and found in many processed foods, these are toxic and have no health benefits whatsoever.

Eat fruit and vegetables You can eat as much salad, and steamed, stir-fried or baked vegetables as you like (within the specified meals), as long as they don't have added dressing or oil (apart from the amount specified in the plan). You can add as much lemon juice, balsamic vinegar or apple cider vinegar as you like. Fruit is also included in healthy, specified portions in the plan.

Eat slowly and chew thoroughly Take time to enjoy and savour all your food (meals and snacks). Chewing food properly aids efficient digestion, stops you from overeating and reduces any uncomfortable bloating you may experience from eating too quickly.

Drink plenty of water As well as keeping yourself hydrated throughout the day, make sure you drink 1–2 glasses of water before *every* meal or snack you have. If you have difficulty drinking enough plain water (around 2 litres a day), herbal teas, green tea (hot or iced) or lemon in hot water are all just as good.

No sugary soft drinks or fruit juice The reason for this is explained in Chapter 3.

Weigh yourself Weigh yourself first thing in the morning, after you've gone to the toilet, without any clothes on. During the attack phase I advised you to weigh yourself every day, just for the first four weeks. The theory behind this, and why it is beneficial for weight loss, is explained in Chapter 11, which introduces you to the attack phase. After the first four weeks, once you're on the lifestyle phase, you should weigh yourself in the same way, once a week.

Start your morning with a mug of warm water and apple cider vinegar Even better than warm water and lemon – often promoted as the healthiest way to start the day – I advise kicking off the morning with a mug of warm water and apple cider vinegar. Use a tablespoon of apple cider vinegar – a wonder food with lots of healing properties – in a mug of warm water. The drink will hydrate you and cleanse your digestive system. More effective than a probiotic, it's the perfect way to set your body up for its daily food intake ahead, as well as helping to prevent bloating. Even though it's a vinegar, it actually neutralises acid, and puts your body in a good pH balance so that your internal system works well. It can also kill bad stomach and intestine bacteria, and promotes good gut bacteria.

Have a big hot drink with your breakfast (and at mid-morning) This provides a warm, comforting start to the day which, combined with a good breakfast, leaves you feeling satisfied for the day ahead. You can drink tea, coffee, or herbal or green tea. Stick to skimmed, soya or almond milk, with no added sugar; sweeteners, such as stevia or xylitol, are allowed with no restriction (see page 46).

A word on caffeine While excess caffeine is obviously no good, caffeine from good-quality coffee (without added sugar, syrups or whipped cream) is packed full of antioxidants and has been shown to have tremendous health benefits. When consumed before a workout, it has also been shown to boost performance and stamina while exercising. Stick to a maximum of two coffees a day, preferably early in the day, not in the late afternoon or evening, so as not to disrupt your sleep.

Limit (but don't shun) alcohol There are many health benefits to alcohol as long as it's consumed in moderation and you stick to the right choices. Drink no more than three glasses a week during the attack phase, and a maximum of one glass per night (up to seven drinks a week) once on the lifestyle phase. Stick to the drinks listed in the 'drink this' (or occasionally 'be careful') column of the beverages section in tables (see page 27). This limit will help you lose weight, clear your head and improve your energy levels, without making you cut out alcohol completely. For more details on alcohol consumption, see Chapter 9).

Don't give up or get despondent We're all human and have our 'ups and downs'. While you are aiming to achieve good discipline with your food choices, The Food Effect healthy-eating lifestyle is not intended to starve or deprive you. If you do slip up, it's not the end of the world. Don't feel as though you've failed and then set yourself back with a total binge fest – just accept it and move on.

Enjoy your Food Effect journey Remember that as long as you continue to be consistent in the process, you *will* reap the benefits and get fantastic results.

Tips to ensure your healthy-lifestyle changes last

Change your mindset Don't think of The Food Effect healthy-eating and weight-loss plan as a 'diet'– something you 'go on' and eventually 'go off'. Reframe this as a new way of life. That way, when or if you do 'slip up', you'll be less likely to give up and get despondent because you'll realise that one or two meals (or even days), of not-too-perfect eating won't undo your overall commitment to a healthy lifestyle; you'll just get straight back on to your normal healthy routine afterwards. Also, while many people start out a healthy-eating plan with a specific goal weight in mind, the *real* goal is to be healthy – weight loss is just a fantastic side effect. So when you do reach your weight-loss goal, you won't shift back to your old habits because it's all about feeling great.

Be realistic If you love a sweet treat or chocolate, for example, don't try to stick to a long-term healthy-eating plan thinking you'll never have these things again. Instead, be realistic and allow for special occasions, indulgences or controlled amounts of your 'vice' food – perhaps switching to a healthier version of it (such as 70 per cent dark chocolate instead of poor-quality, highly processed milk chocolate).

Set manageable goals By doing the opposite (that is, being unrealistic), you just set yourself up for failure and worse, *feeling* like a failure, and are thus more likely to give up altogether. If the thought of eating a bowl of healthy greens makes you nauseous, make changes in small increments; for example, by adding one serving of fresh vegetables a day, until you're ready to push for more.

Team up Research has shown that dieters are more successful when they have support. That may involve partnering with a friend to do The Food Effect diet, or asking family members to encourage you and provide support. If you feel that your eating habits are tied to emotional issues (not an uncommon problem), such as loneliness, depression and so on, consider seeking help for those issues too.

Prepare, prepare, prepare This is the golden rule of successful healthy eating habits. The more you think ahead and take a few moments to plan and prepare your food, the more likely and easier it will be for you to enjoy healthy and tasty food, and the less likely you will be to make unhealthy choices when going about your day, rushed in the moment. Think ahead about the food and meals you intend to eat, and make sure you have the right things on hand (you now have plenty of perfect examples and suggestions). If you're constantly on the go, that will be no excuse for unhealthy eating – just make sure you have grab-and-go options always on hand (The Food Effect plan and meal options provide plenty of easy suggestions).

Perfect your shopping list As I said at the start of this chapter, if you buy good food, you'll eat good food. Similarly, if you don't buy junk food and keep it stocked at home, you'll be less likely to eat junk food altogether. Everyone in your home will benefit from this one, too. See kitchen staples on pages 245–249 for the basics on what to have stocked.

Treat yourself With non-food rewards. Choose small rewards for reaching your goals along the way (and bigger ones for bigger goals). Try to choose a treat for yourself that will further enhance your 'feel-good' lifestyle (such as a massage or an indulgent pampering product), or perhaps even something that will fuel it further (like some stylish workout clothing you've been eyeing).

Make it enjoyable Make your healthful Food Effect lifestyle fun and enjoyable. Try new healthy recipes, share them with friends or cook for others. Get ideas online via social media – there are loads of great nutrition blogs out there. To start with, check out www.thefoodeffect.co.uk for ongoing cooking inspiration and all the latest in nutrition. Make sure you follow The Food Effect on Facebook, Twitter and Instagram **@thefoodeffectdr** for your daily dose of inspiration.

REFERENCES

Chapter 2

Steinberg, D.M., Bennett, G.G., Askew, S., Tate, D.F., 'Weighing every day matters: daily weighing improves weight loss and adoption of weight control behaviors', *Journal of Academy of Nutrition and Dietetics*, 114(4) (2015), pp. 511–518.

Chapter 3

Hyun-seok Kim, 'Prevalence of celiac appears steady but followers of gluten-free diet increase', *JAMA Internal Medicine*, 6 September 2016.

Chapter 4

Kritchevsky, S.B. and Kritchevsky D., 'Egg consumption and coronary heart disease: an epidemiologic overview', *Journal of the American College of Nutrition*, 19 (2000), pp. 549S–555S; McNamara, D.J. , 'The impact of egg limitations on coronary heart disease risk: do the numbers add up?', *Journal of the American College of Nutrition* 19 (2000), pp. 540S–548S.

Memisoglu A., Hu F. B., Hankinson S. E., Manson J. E., De Vivo I., Willett W. C., Hunter D. J., 'Interaction between a peroxisome proliferator-activated receptor gamma gene polymorphism and dietary fat intake in relation to body mass', *Human Molecular Genetics*, 12(22) (2003), pp. 2923–2929.

Esselstyn C. B. Jr., Gendy G., Doyle J., Golubic M., Roizen M. F., 'A way to reverse CAD?' *The Journal of Family Practice,* 63(7) (2014), pp. 356–364b.

Chapter 5

Mingyang Song, 'Eating more plant protein associated with lower risk of death', *JAMA Internal Medicine*, 1 August 2016.

Bujnowski D., Xun P., Daviglus, M. L., Van Horn, L., He K., Stamler J., 'Longitudinal association between animal and vegetable protein intake and obesity among men in the United States: the Chicago Western Electric Study', *Journal of the American Dietetic Association,* 111(8) (2011), pp. 1150–1155.e1.

Wang X., Lin X., Ouyang Y. Y., Liu J., Zhao G., Pan A., Hu F. B., 'Red and processed meat consumption and mortality: dose-response meta-analysis of prospective cohort studies', *Public Health Nutrition,* 19(5) (2016), pp. 893–905.

Pan A., Sun Q., Bernstein A. M., Schulze M. B., Manson J. E., Stampfer M. J., Willett W. C., Hu F. B., 'Red meat consumption and mortality: results from 2 prospective cohort studies', *Archives of Internal Medicine,* 172(7) (2012), pp. 555–563.

Lagiou P., Sandin S., Weiderpass E., Lagiou A., Mucci L., Trichopoulos D., Adami H. O., ' Low carbohydrate–high protein diet and mortality in a cohort of Swedish women', *Journal of Internal Medicine,* 261(4) (2007), pp. 366–374.

Fung T. T., van Dam R. M., Hankinson S. E, Stampfer M., Willett W. C., Hu F. B., 'Low-carbohydrate diets and all-cause and cause-specific mortality: two cohort studies', *Annals of Internal Medicine,* 153(5) (2010), pp. 289–298.

Pan A., Sun Q., Bernstein A. M., Manson J. E., Willett W. C., Hu F.B., 'Changes in red meat consumption and subsequent risk of type 2 diabetes mellitus: three cohorts of US men and women', *JAMA Internal Medicine,* 173(14) (2013), pp. 1328–1335.

Morris M. C., Evans D. A, Bienias J. L., Tangney C. C., Bennett D. A., Aggarwal N., Schneider J., Wilson R. S., 'Dietary fats and the risk of incident Alzheimer disease', *Archives of Neurology,* 60(2) (2003), pp. 194–200.

Richman E. L, Kenfield S. A., Stampfer M. J., Giovannucci E. L., Zeisel S. H., Willett W. C., Chan J. M., 'Choline intake and risk of lethal prostate cancer: incidence and survival', *American Journal of Clinical Nutrition*, 96(4) (2012), pp. 855–863.

Ornish D., Magbanua M. J., Weidner G., Weinberg V., Kemp C., Green C., Mattie M. D., Marlin R., Simko J., Shinohara K., Haqq C. M., Carroll P. R., 'Changes in prostate gene expression in men undergoing an intensive nutrition and lifestyle intervention', *Proceedings of the National Academy of Sciences USA*, 105(24) (2008), pp. 8369–8374.

Parazzini, F., Viganò, P., Candiani, M., Fedele, L., 'Diet and endometriosis risk: A literature review', *American Journal of Obstetrics and Gynecology*, 26(4) (2013), pp. 323–336.

Lewis S. J., Heaton K. W., Oakey R. E. and McGarrigle H. H., 'Lower serum oestrogen concentrations associated with faster intestinal transit', *British Journal of Cancer*, 76(3) (1997), pp. 395–400.

Alexander, D.D., Morimoto, L.M., Mink, P.J., and Cushing, C.A., 'A review and meta-analysis of red and processed meat consumption and breast cancer', *Cambridge University Press*, 23(2) (2010), pp. 349–365.

Ping-Ping Bao, Xiao-Ou Shu, Ying Zheng, Hui Cai, Zhi-Xian Ruan, Kai Gu, Yinghao Su, Yu-Tang Gao, Wei Zheng and Wei Lu, 'Fruit, vegetable, and animal food intake and breast cancer risk by hormone receptor status', *Nutriton and Cancer*, 64(6) (2012), pp. 806–819.

National Cancer Institute, 'Chemicals in meat cooked at high temperatures and cancer risk', https://www.cancer.gov/about-cancer/causes-prevention/risk/diet/cooked-meats-fact-sheet

Frattaroli J., Weidner G., Merritt-Worden T. A., Frenda S., Ornish D., 'Angina pectoris and atherosclerotic risk factors in the multisite cardiac lifestyle intervention programme', *American Journal of Cardiology*, 101(7) (2008), pp. 911–918.

Chapter 6

de Gaetano, G., 'Mediterranean diet associated with lower risk of early death in cardiovascular disease patients', *European Society of Cardiology*, 29 August 2016.

Morris M. C. , Evans D. A., Bienias J. L., Tangney C. C., Bennett D. A., Aggarwal N., Schneider J., Wilson R. S., 'Dietary fats and the risk of incident Alzheimer disease', *Archives of Neurology,* 60(2) (2003), pp. 194–200.

Endocrine Society, 'To reduce body fat, eating less fat may be more effective than eating less carbohydrate', *Science Daily,* 5 March 2015. www.sciencedaily.com/releases/2015/03/150305151834.htm

Memisoglu A., Hu F. B., Hankinson S. E., Manson J. E., De Vivo I., Willett W. C., Hunter D. J., 'Interaction between a peroxisome proliferator-activated receptor gamma gene polymorphism and dietary fat intake in relation to body mass', *Human Molecular Genetics,*12(22) (2003), pp. 2923–2929.

Chapter 7

Soutschek, A., Ruff, C.C., Strombach, T., Kalenscher, T., and Tobler, P.N., 'Brain stimulation reveals crucial role of overcoming self-centeredness in self-control', *Science Advances*, 2(10) (2016), e1600992. DOI: 10.1126/sciadv.1600992.

Chapter 9

Berkey, C. S. et al., 'Weight gain in older adolescent females: the internet, sleep, coffee, and alcohol', *Journal of Pediatrics,* 153(5) (2008), p. 639.

Gruchow, H. W. et al., 'Alcohol consumption, nutrient intake and relative body weight among US adults', *American Journal of Clinical Nutrition* 1985; 42: pp. 289–295.

Arif, A. A. and Rohrer, J. E., 'Patterns of alcohol drinking and its association with obesity: data from the third national health and nutrition examination survey 1988–1994', *BMC Public Health,* 5(5) (2005), p. 126.

Wang, L. et al., 'Alcohol consumption, weight gain, and risk of becoming overweight in middle-aged and older women', *Archives of Internal Medicine,* 170(5) (2010), pp. 453–461.

Lahti-Koski, M. et al., 'Associations of body mass index and obesity with physical activity, food choices, alcohol intake, and smoking in the 1982–1997 FINRISK studies', *American Journal of Clinical Nutrition,* 75(5) (2002), pp. 809–817.

Chapter 10

Malhotra A., Noakes T., Phinney S., 'It is time to bust the myth of physical inactivity and obesity: you cannot outrun a bad diet', *British Journal of Sports Medicine,* 49 (2015), pp. 967–968.

Pereira, A., Huddleston, D., Brickman A. et al., 'An in vivo correlate of exercise-induced neurogenesis in the adult dentate gyrus', *Proceedings of the National Academy of Sciences USA,* 104(13) (2007), pp. 5638–5643.

Ornish D., Lin J., Chan J. M., Epel E., Kemp C., Weidner G., Marlin R., Frenda S. J., Magbanua M. J., Daubenmier J., Estay I., Hills N.K., Chainani-Wu N., Carroll P.R., Blackburn E. H., 'Effect of comprehensive lifestyle changes on telomerase activity and telomere length in men with biopsy-proven low-risk prostate cancer: 5-year follow-up of a descriptive pilot study', *Lancet Oncology,* 14(11) (2013), pp. 1112–1120.

Frattaroli J., Weidner G., Merritt-Worden T. A., Frenda S., Ornish D., 'Angina pectoris and atherosclerotic risk factors in the multisite cardiac lifestyle intervention program', *American Journal of Cardiology,* 101(7) (2008), pp. 911–918.

'Everyone should take vitamin D pills, doctors warn', *The Times,* Thursday, 21 July 2016.

Chapter 11

Steinberg, D.M., Bennett, G.G., Askew, S., Tate, D.F., 'Weighing every day matters: daily weighing improves weight loss and adoption of weight control behaviors', *Journal of Academy of Nutrition and Dietetics*, 114(4) (2015), pp. 511–518.

INDEX

ACKNOWLEDGEMENTS

My deepest thanks to my most incredible literary agent Heather Holden-Brown of hhb Agency, and the amazing Cara Armstrong. Heather, you had faith in me from day one, when this book was just an idea in my head. Your constant guidance, support and unwavering encouragement enabled me to make my dreams a reality.

Thank you to everyone at Little, Brown for making this book everything that it is. A special thank-you to Zoe Bohm and Jillian Stewart, who gave me invaluable editorial guidance and supported me every step along the way. You are both beyond thorough and talented at everything you do.

Thank you to Tracey Winwood for co-ordinating and putting together the cover design.

Thank you to Liron Weissman and Avia Soloman for your incredible skills!

Thank you to my amazing mum and dad – there are no words to express my love for you both or my gratitude for everything you have done, and continue to do, for me. You are my role models in every aspect of life, and have supported me in everything I do since the day I was born. Thank you to my amazing siblings, Bruce, Hayley and Adina; siblings-in-law and family and friends for always being there for me. I love you all so much.

Thank you to the love of my life, my husband Jeff. There are no words to express how much I love and adore you, and how much you brighten up my life. You encourage and support me with my work and ambitions, and are always there to inspire me to achieve my dreams. Thank you for being my rock in everything I do.

Finally, thank you so much to all my clients, past and present – I'd never have gained all the knowledge and insight into successful weight loss and how people deal with eating, dieting and life, without all of you. You've all inspired me so much!

Thank you so much. M xx